No Miracle Cures
A Multifactorial Guide to Stuttering Therapy

Thomas David Kehoe

Owner, Casa Futura Technologies

Member, American Speech-Language Hearing Association

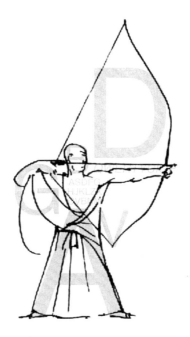

University College Press

616.8554
Keh

Publisher Cataloging-In-Publication Data
Kehoe, Thomas David
No Miracle Cures/Thomas David Kehoe
Includes index.

ISBN-10 0-9657181-6-6   SAN 299-2566
ISBN-13 978-0-9657181-6-5
Library of Congress Control Number: (applied for May 31, 2006)
Library of Congress Subject Heading: RC424 .K45 2006
Dewey Decimal Classification: 616.8554
BASIC: MED007000 MEDICAL/Audiology & Speech Pathology
BIC Standard Subject Category: MQMF

Printed in the United States of America

Published by   University College Press, an imprint of
Casa Futura Technologies
720 31st St
Boulder, CO 80303-2402
(303) 417-9752
http://www.casafuturatech.com/Books/

TABLE OF CONTENTS

INTRODUCTION 1
What stuttering is, and the factors that contribute to stuttering

ANTI-STUTTERING DEVICES.. 11
From immediate fluency to long-term carryover

FLUENCY SHAPING THERAPY 28
Learning to speak with relaxed speech-production muscles

BEYOND FLUENCY SHAPING... 57
Making fluent speech automatic and effortless

RESPONDING TO STRESS 76
Good stress, bad stress; how stuttering reduces stress

ANTI-STUTTERING MEDICATIONS 100
And anti-depressants that increase stuttering

PSYCHOLOGICAL ISSUES.. 107
Denial, anger, and speech-related fears and anxieties

CHILDHOOD STUTTERING.. 118
Preschool, school-age, teenagers

FAMOUS PEOPLE WHO STUTTER.. 139
Actors, singers, athletes, writers, political and business leaders, more

STUTTERING SUPPORT GROUPS 153
You're not alone; support group activities

STUTTERING AT WORK.. 160
How to handle job interviews; the Americans with Disabilities Act

LISTENER REACTIONS 165
What happened when I asked listeners about my stuttering

OTHER FLUENCY DISORDERS 170
Cluttering, neurogenic and psychogenic stuttering, spastic dysphonia

RECOMMENDED BOOKS 173

PRACTICE WORD LISTS 175

ACKNOWLEDGEMENTS

Thanks to Greg Snyder, Tom Morrow, John Harrison, Richard Harkness, Nancy Peske, Alice B. Kehoe, and Mary Anne Siderits; and to Kate Hawley for the cover design.

Note

80% of adult stutterers are male so this book refers to stutterers as *he*. 93% of speech-language pathologists are female so this book refers to SLPs as *she*.

Introduction

I stuttered severely. I needed an hour to say what a non-stutterer could say in five minutes. I could block on a word for five minutes.

My speech wasn't just slow. I jerked my head, rolled my eyes, and my body shook in spasms. Some listeners asked if I needed medical attention. More often they laughed at me.

Worst, my speech was incomprehensible. Listeners guessed what I was trying to say, usually wrong. Or they ignored me and walked away.

I'm now forty-four. People ask me to speak at events. I perform acting and stand-up comedy. In stressful conversations I sound confident and relaxed. And I still stutter.

Wait a minute! How can I stutter and have listeners say that it's a pleasure to hear me speak? Let me tell you about some other stutterers.

Demosthenes stuttered, and became the greatest orator of ancient Greece. Winston Churchill and Aneurin Bevan were the best orators in the British Parliament in the 1930s and 1940s. Both men stuttered.

James Earl Jones, John Stossel, Bruce Willis, Nicholas Brendan, Mel Tillis, Carly Simon, and hundreds of other actors, singers, politicians, and business leaders have stuttered.

Not many paraplegics win marathons. Few blind persons become famous painters. Not a lot of deaf persons are great musicians.

But stuttering is a different kind of disability. Treating stuttering trains you to improve your speech. You'll learn to handle stressful situations calmly. You'll learn to relax your breathing and your voice. Years after reading this book, you'll look back over many life successes and say that stuttering was a gift.

Developmental Disorders

Stuttering isn't a physical disorder. It's not a psychological disorder. Stuttering is a *developmental disorder*. The primary reason that adults stutter is that we stuttered as children.

Children grow up in a certain order. They crawl before they walk. They walk before they run. They run before they ride bicycles. They ride bicycles before they borrow your car keys.

Usually. Some children walk before they crawl. My three-year-old nephew borrows my car all the time. Just joking. I don't own a car.

At each stage of physical development, a child's brain develops too. For example, crawling helps the child develop communication between the left and right hemispheres of his brain. If all goes well, the child's physical, neurological, and psychological systems develop together.

A small, sometimes imperceptible, developmental misstep in early childhood can nudge a child off the normal developmental track. The child then grows on an abnormal developmental track. A minor problem can develop into a major disability as the child grows up.

Language-Learning Impairment

Another developmental communications disorder is better understood than stuttering. Children with *language-learning impairment* (LLI, also called *specific language impairment* or SLI) experience difficulties in understanding and producing spoken language despite normal intelligence, normal hearing, and normal opportunities to learn language.[1]

LLI results when a child can't hear the difference between short duration speech sounds. The difference between /b/ and /d/ sounds occurs within a few milliseconds (thousands of a second). Some children's brains' auditory processing isn't fast enough to hear fast speech sounds. To these kids, "bad" and "dad" are the same word, "bug" and "dug" are the same, and so are "buck" and "duck." This is a form of *central auditory processing disorder*, or CAPD.

You'd think this would be a minor problem. After all, you know the difference between "sew" and "so." But it's not a minor problem. These children develop speech slower than other children. Slow speech development causes them to miss other developmental stages. Their grammar develops poorly. Listeners have difficulty understanding these children's speech. These children understand the difference between boys and girls, but interchange "he" and "she." They mix up past, present, and future tense.

Then these children are labeled mentally retarded, even though they're normal or even excel at non-language activities (e.g., building with Legos). They're put into special ed classes, with children who really are mentally retarded.

The children miss more developmental stages. As adults, these individuals may be unable to read, or have poor social skills, or be unable to work at more than menial jobs.

Ten years ago a treatment was developed for LLI. These children can distinguish /b/ from /d/ if the words are slowed down. Children with LLI now play a computer game that trains them to hear the difference between short-duration speech sounds.[2]

When their auditory dysfunction is corrected, the children develop normally. The children usually catch up with their peers, e.g., advancing four reading grade levels in six months.

Analogously, children's brains are like a railroad going from New York to Los Angeles. A little dysfunction can bump a child onto a sidetrack. The sidetrack may start out only a few feet from the main track, but twenty years later he's lost somewhere in South America. Treatment is like giving the child a shove back onto the main railroad track. The child then zooms ahead to catch up with his peers.

Factors that Contribute to Stuttering

Functional brain scans show three abnormalities during stuttering[3]:

- Overactive motor (muscle movement) areas.

- Underactive auditory processing areas. [4]
- Speech-related brain areas that typically have left-hemisphere dominance in fluent speakers are active bilaterally or with right-hemisphere dominance in stutterers.

Anatomical brain scans of stutterers have found abnormalities in the left hemisphere superior temporal gyrus (the location of the primary auditory cortex and Wernicke's area, associated with speech and language processing[5]) and Rolandic operculum (the location of Broca's area, associated with speech production[6]).

All brain scan studies have examined adult male stutterers. We don't know whether some children are born with these abnormalities, which then cause stuttering; or if children have normal brain activity and anatomy when they begin stuttering, and stuttering causes their brains to develop (grow) abnormally.

These results suggest that stuttering doesn't have a single cause, but rather several factors contribute to stuttering. Two of the three functional brain abnormalities correspond roughly to treatments for stuttering; the third is more ambiguous.

Speech Motor Overactivity

Speech motor overactivity associated with stuttering includes overtense respiration (breathing); vocal folds; and lips, jaws, and tongues (articulators). These overtense muscles lock or fail to coordinate, making speech impossible. *Fluency shaping therapy* (page 28) trains stutterers to speak with relaxed speech production muscles, to counteract our overactive speech motor activity. You learn to consciously relax your breathing; vocal folds; and lips, jaw, and tongue. That's relatively easy. The following chapter ("Beyond Fluency Shaping," page 57) is about the more difficult task of making this fluent speech automatic and effortless.

The neurotransmitter dopamine is related to motor activity. Dopamine antagonist medications diminish stuttering. These treatments are presented in the chapter "Anti-Stuttering Medications" (page 100).

Auditory Processing Underactivity
Like LLI, stuttering may be related to a central auditory processing disorder.

Changes in how stutterers hear our voice, such as choral speech and anti-stuttering devices (page 11) appear to correct the auditory processing underactivity associated with stuttering.

Right Hemisphere Lateralization
The anomalous lateralization doesn't yet have a clear explanation. The right frontal operculum may relate to production and perception of vocal fundamental frequency[7], which is a key part of fluency shaping therapy (e.g., "easy onsets" or "gentle onsets").

But similar frontal operculum activity is seen in Tourette's syndrome[8] (see pages 100, 122), so perhaps this brain activity relates to features common to both disorders. For example, both disorders tend to decrease when a person is relaxed, but increase when the person experiences certain types of stress. The chapter "Responding to Stress" (page 76) describes how our brains unconsciously select different ways of speaking (speech motor parameters) depending on environmental cues. That chapter also presents treatments to help you make this process conscious, so that you can choose to speak fluently in situations that previously caused you to stutter.

The brain's right hemisphere is generally associated with emotions (the left hemisphere is associated more with logic and reasoning). Possibly the abnormal right-hemisphere activity indicates emotional activity associated with stuttering. For some individuals, speech-related fears and anxieties are more disabling than their physical stuttering. Some individuals use stuttering as an excuse for deeper psychological problems. Some individuals obsessively try to hide their stuttering, e.g., counterproductively refusing to go to speech therapy for fear that someone may see them entering the speech clinic. The chapter "Psychological Issues" (page 107) addresses these feelings, attitudes, and other emotions.

Multifactorial Treatment and Additional Factors

No single stuttering therapy works for every stutterer. Treating stuttering requires a *multifactorial* approach—different treatments for each factor. And different stutterers may have more or less of each factor, so different stutterers respond better or worse to different treatments.

Speech-language pathologists usually treat one or more of three factors: speech motor skills, stress management, and/or psychological counseling. Electronic anti-stuttering devices treat one or two factors: auditory processing and/or speech motor skills. Dopamine-antagonist medications treat one factor. You may have to go to several speech clinics, and possibly buy an electronic device or get a medication prescription, to treat all of the factors that contribute to your stuttering.

I expect that additional stuttering factors will be discovered. Future advances will also include be treatments for co-existing conditions. E.g., a child with stuttering and phonological dysfunction will be treated differently than a child with stuttering and ADHD. An adult with stuttering and social phobia will be treated differently from an outgoing mentally retarded adult who stutters.

What is Stuttering?

Speech begins with breathing, also called *respiration*. Your lungs fill with air, more air than you would inhale if you weren't talking. You expand your upper chest and your diaphragm (belly) to get all this air in. Your lung pressure and respiration muscle tension increase.

Next, you release air through your throat, past your vocal folds (also called *vocal cords*). Your vocal folds are a pair of small muscles in your larynx. If you tense these muscles slightly, and release a little air, your vocal folds vibrate. This is called *phonation*. It's also called the *fundamental frequency* of your voice. If you place your fingers on the front of your throat, then hum or talk, you can feel your vocal folds vibrating.

Adult men vibrate their vocal folds about 125 Hz (125 times per second). Women vibrate their vocal folds about 200 Hz. Children's voices are even higher. This is too fast for your brain to control. Vocal fold vibration is the only muscle activity that your brain doesn't directly control. Instead, phonation results from the coordination of respiration muscles to release air with slight tensing of your vocal fold muscles.

The key word in that last sentence was *coordination*. Stuttering is largely a disorder of poorly coordinated speech production muscles.

If you tense your vocal folds too much, you block off your throat and stop air from escaping your lungs. This is a good when lifting heavy weights. By blocking your larynx and tensing your respiration muscles, you increase lung pressure, which strengthens your chest and you can lift more weight. Similarly, tires inflated to high pressure can carry a heavier car. But that's what stutterers do when they talk, and it's not a good idea.

The space in your throat above your larynx is called the *pharynx*. Above your pharynx are your oral and nasal cavities. These spaces create vocal resonation. This is like the echoing of a cathedral or tunnel. The unique shape of these spaces makes each of our voices sound unique.

Your jaw and lips and tongue, collectively called the *articulation muscles*, modify your voice into intelligible speech.

Vowels and *voiced* consonants (such as /b/ and /d/) are produced by your vocal folds, and modified by your articulation muscles (jaw, lips, tongue).

Other consonants are *voiceless*, such as /p/ and /t/, produced by your articulation muscles modifying airflow, without your vocal folds vibrating. When you whisper, you don't vibrate your vocal folds. You just modify airflow with your articulation muscles.

Speech requires coordination of over 100 muscles. The average person speaks about 150 words per minute. Each word requires a different configuration of most of those muscles. Speech is our most complex neuromuscular activity.

Core Stuttering Behaviors

- *Disordered breathing*, including antagonism between abdominal (belly) and thoracic (upper chest) respiratory muscles; complete cessation of breathing, and interrupting exhalation with inhalation.
- *Disordered vocal folds*, including high levels of muscle activity or muscle tension; poor laryngeal muscle timing, such as starting phonation too late or holding tension too long; and poor coordination of laryngeal muscles, e.g., incompatible contractions of opposing muscles.
- *Disordered articulation*, including dysfunctions of the lips, jaw, and tongue in stuttering. In general, stutterers place their articulators in the right positions (in contrast to other speech disorders such as lisping), but time the movements wrong.
- *Low-frequency tremors* in the neck, jaw, and lip muscles of adult stutterers. These are found to a lesser extent in older children, and not found in young children who stutter.[9]

Secondary Stuttering Behaviors

Secondary stuttering behaviors are unrelated to speech production:

- Physical movements such as eye-blinking, forehead wrinkling, sudden exhaustion of breath, frowning, or nostril quivering.
- Gross (large) muscle movements such as head jerks or slapping one's thigh in an attempt to release a vocal fold block or other overtense speech-production muscle.
- Fear of certain words or sounds, avoidance of feared words, substitution of another word, or postponement of a feared word by adding pauses or filler words.
- Interjected "starter" sounds and words, such as "um," "ah," "you know," or "in other words."
- Repeating a sentence or phrase "to get a running start."
- Vocal abnormalities to prevent stuttering, such as speaking

in a rapid monotone, affecting an accent, or using odd inflections.

- Looking away, not maintaining eye contact.
- Articulating an unrelated sound, e.g., forming a /t/ sound when trying to say /s/.

Secondary behaviors may help you get around stuttering at first, but then lose their effectiveness. The secondary behavior is then retained out of habit.

Incidence and Prevalence

About 2.5% of preschool children stutter now (prevalence).[10] The incidence of preschool stuttering is about 5%. In other words, about one in twenty of children stutter at some point in childhood.

Less than 1% of adults stutter. 0.73%, or about one in 135 adults, was the figure found in a recent study.[11] That suggests that about two million Americans stutter. On the other hand:

- The largest stuttering therapy program, the National Center for Stuttering, has treated about 10,000 stutterers. The second-largest stuttering therapy program, the Hollins Communication Research Institute, has treated about 5,000 stutterers. [12]
- Other stuttering therapy programs are much smaller. Less than 400 speech-language pathologists are board-certified Fluency Specialists. Most treat only a handful of adult stutterers each year.
- About 2500 Edinburgh Masker anti-stuttering devices were sold in the United States in the 1980s. My company has each sold about three thousand anti-stuttering devices.
- The National Stuttering Association has about 2500 members. The biggest stuttering support e-mail list has about three thousand members.

How many stutterers have you met, out of thousands of people you hear talking every year? The number of adult stutterers may be closer to 20,000, not two million.

A Wikibook and a Discussion Forum

I put a version of this book on the Wikibooks website:

http://en.wikibooks.org/wiki/Speech-Language_Pathology/Stuttering

The wikibook is longer than *No Miracle Cures*. With zero cost for paper or printing, there was no reason to leave out material of interest to only a few individuals, e.g., stuttering therapy for mentally retarded individuals.

The wikibook includes hyperlinks to related material, e.g., a link to an article about Tourette's syndrome.

The wikibook includes criticism. In *No Miracle Cures*, if I felt that a popular theory was wrong, I left it out. In the wikibook, I included the theory, and then detailed why it's wrong.

The wikibook is interactive. You can add material, correct my mistakes, or even edit any part of the book. What matters isn't whether I got every fact right or referenced every study. What matters is that you can fix my mistakes.

Some chapters are set up to encourage reader participation. The chapter "How We Treat Stuttering" encourages speech-language pathologists to describe what they do. The chapter "What Worked For Me" encourages stutterers to add material.

And every page has a discussion area. You just click on a tab to ask questions or make comments.

And *No Miracle Cures* has its own discussion forum. Just go to

http://www.casafuturatech.com

and click on "Discussion Forum." That's the place to ask any questions you have while reading this book.

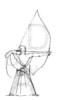

Anti-Stuttering Devices

Our ears hear sounds. The *central auditory processing* area of our brains processes those perceived sounds into useful information, such as words. Central auditory processing disorder (CAPD) is not a single disorder but rather is an umbrella term for anything wrong with how our brains process auditory information. A wide variety of disorders seem to have a CAPD component, including ADHD and language disorders.[13] CAPD is not a hearing disorder, i.e., a person with CAPD usually has nothing wrong with his or her ears.

Brain scans have found that adult stutterers appear to have abnormal underactivity in their central auditory processing area. What's wrong with adult stutterers' auditory processing is unknown. If I had to guess, I'd say that stutterers have something wrong with how we hear our own voices. One study suggested that adult stutterers have an inability to integrate auditory and somatic processing,[14] i.e., comparing what we hear ourselves saying to how we feel our muscles moving.

If this is true, then stuttering is one of many *sensory integration disorders* (SID) that originate in childhood. Perhaps stuttering therapy should include exercises to train one to listen to one's speech and feel one's muscles moving.

Other CAPD Symptoms

I have other symptoms associated with mild CAPD. I prefer to watch movies with the subtitles on. I can't "pick up" foreign languages by ear; I have to study a written language before I can hear words, and then only if spoken slowly. If there's background noise, such as wind, I can't understand what people are saying.

Other symptoms of CAPD include sensitivity to certain noises; difficulty identifying the direction of sounds; difficulty following multi-step directions, especially if given in one sentence; and reading, spelling, and speech problems.

Altered Auditory Feedback

Changing how stutterers hear their voices improves fluency. This can be done in many ways:

- Speaking in chorus with another person.
- Hearing your voice in headphones distorted.
- Hearing a synthesized sound in headphones mimicking your phonation (masking auditory feedback, or MAF).
- Hearing your voice in headphones delayed a fraction of a second (delayed auditory feedback, or DAF).
- Hearing your voice in headphones shifted higher or lower in pitch (frequency-shifted auditory feedback, or FAF).

These phenomena are called *altered auditory feedback.* No brain scans have looked at stutterers' auditory processing while speaking with altered auditory feedback.[15] Hypothetically, introducing errors targeted at the area that integrates auditory and somatic processing increases blood flow to that area, increasing activity level to normal.

In other words, hearing what you're saying out of sync with what you feel your muscles doing raises a red flag. The red flag is raised in an area that's abnormally underactive in stutterers. It's like a poor little overlooked village suddenly saying, "The British are coming! Eureka! There's gold in them thar hills! We've struck oil! Aliens have landed!"

Picture wagon trains, locomotives, and paratroopers descending on this sleepy little burg. In brain terms, more blood flows to this area.

The errors must *not* raise red flags in other brain areas, such as language processing. I built a device that, when you walked up to Fred and said, "Hi, Fred," the device whispered in your ear, "Hi, Steve." It didn't improve fluency. It stopped everyone—stutterers and non-stutterers—from talking.

Non-stutterers can't tolerate altered auditory feedback. I've amused many non-stutterers by putting an anti-stuttering device on them and telling them to count to twenty. Most can't get to ten. They repeat or skip numbers, or giggle uncontrollably, then rip the headphones off.

If my hypothesis is correct, then altered auditory feedback increases blood flow to non-stutterers' auditory/somatic integration area, raising activity to an abnormally high level. Too much activity is as bad as not enough activity. Interestingly, the effects of too much activity in this area are somewhat like stuttering—repeating words and unexpected silent pauses.

Planum Temporale Abnormality and DAF

The planum temporale (PT) is an anatomical feature in the auditory temporal brain region. Typically people have a larger PT on the left side of their brains, and smaller PT on the right side (leftward asymmetry). A brain scan study found that stutterers have the opposite: their right PT is larger than their left PT (rightward asymmetry).[16]

A second study found that stutterers with this abnormal rightward asymmetry had significantly improved fluency with DAF, but stutterers with the normal leftward asymmetry didn't improve with DAF.[17] The study also found that stutterers with this abnormal rightward asymmetry stuttered more severely than stutterers with the normal leftward asymmetry.

Delayed Auditory Feedback

Delayed auditory feedback (DAF) seems to have two distinct effects, depending on whether the delay is short (25 to 75 milliseconds, or about a twentieth of a second) or long (75-200 milliseconds, or about a tenth of a second).

A short delay immediately reduces stuttering about 70%,[18] without training, mental effort, or abnormally slow or abnormal-sounding speech. You just put on the headphones and talk. Hypothetically, this effect results from correcting a central auditory processing abnormality. While this effect is impressive, it doesn't 100% eliminate stuttering, and the effect goes away when the headphones are removed. A short delay appears to correct one factor in stuttering.

A longer delay induces a slower speaking rate with stretched vowels (continuous phonation) target (page 33). This requires training and sounds abnormally slow and monotonic.

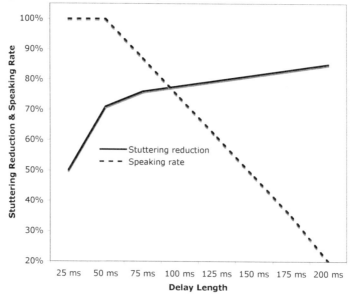

Figure 1: DAF Effectiveness

The chart shows that at normal speaking rates, a short delay can reduce but not eliminate stuttering. A longer delay can reduce stuttering further, at the expense of speaking rate.[19]

Using DAF in Therapy

DAF stuttering therapy begins with training a stutterer to use the slower speaking rate with stretched vowels target, without using DAF. When the stutterer can complete a simple speaking task, such as counting to ten, using this target correctly, then he can use a DAF device. DAF therapy then has several goals:

- To increase the length and complexity of sentences while

using the DAF device to support on-target fluent speech.

- To increase the stress of the speaking situation while using the DAF device to support on-target fluent speech.
- To reduce the need for the DAF device, until the stutterer no longer needs the device.

In other words, the stutterer first uses the DAF device for short phrases in the speech clinic. Typically this is one or two seconds per syllable, with the delay set at 200 milliseconds. He must achieve all fluent speech targets, e.g., all syllables stretched equally, all syllables stretched to one second, no pauses between words, and no dysfluencies.

The stutterer then uses the device in longer conversations in the speech clinic, again achieving all the fluent speech targets. Then he uses the device in more stressful speaking tasks, such as role playing with his speech-language pathologist (page 94).

When the stutterer achieves these goals, then he decreases the delay and increases his speaking rate. But if he has any dysfluencies he goes back to the longer delay and slower speaking rate.

The stutterer can also decrease the volume, and use the device in one ear instead of both ears. He can use the device at the beginning of conversations, and then turn it off when he feels capable of speaking on target with the support of the device. He can discontinue using the device in low-stress conversations; then in medium-stress conversations; and finally reserving the device only for stressful conversations such as public speaking. Eventually he should need the device only occasionally.

Mistakes in DAF Use

Don't use DAF at normal speaking rate with a long delay. If you want to talk at a normal speaking rate, set the DAF delay between 50 and 75 milliseconds.[20] Don't use a delay longer than 75 milliseconds unless you're using closed-loop slow speech (page 37).

I've seen this scenario over and over. A stutterer gets a 50% fluency improvement at 50 milliseconds. He gets a 75% improvement at 75 milliseconds. He sees that the dial goes up to 200 milliseconds. He thinks, "I'll crank up this baby! I'll redline it! I'll turn it up all the way to 200 milliseconds and I'll be 200% fluent!"

200 milliseconds is for speech five to ten times slower than normal. Non-stutterers can't talk normally with a 200-millisecond delay (with rare exceptions due to a linguistic abnormality) but most stutterers are capable of forcing themselves to "tune out" the delay. This appears to be due to our auditory processing underactivity. In other words, if you use DAF incorrectly you may make your auditory processing underactivity worse. This may explain why some stutterers have reported that a DAF device lost effectiveness or "wore off" over time.

Another mistake is to use a DAF device in low-stress situations (such as reading aloud) and expect carryover to high-stress situations. Carryover works the other way. Use an anti-stuttering device in situations in which you stutter, and don't use it in situations where you speak fluently.

Long-Term Effects of DAF

Nine adult stutterers used DAF devices thirty minutes per day, for three months.[21] The thirty minutes consisted of ten minutes reading aloud, a ten-minute conversation with a family member, and a ten-minute telephone call. The subjects received no speech therapy.

The device used was the School DAF, made by Casa Futura Technologies (my company), with a binaural (two ears) headset. The subjects were allowed to set the delay where they wanted. Most selected delays around 100 milliseconds.

At the start of the study (0 months), the subjects stuttered on 37% of words, on average. With the DAF device their stuttering dropped to 10%. In other words, the device improved their fluency about 70%.

Three months later the subjects stuttered on 17% of words, when not using the DAF device. When wearing the DAF device they stuttered on 13% of words.

This shows that, when not wearing the devices, the subjects' stuttering diminished from 37% of words to 17% of words, or a 55% improvement. This is "carryover fluency," that is, the device training users to need the device less and less.

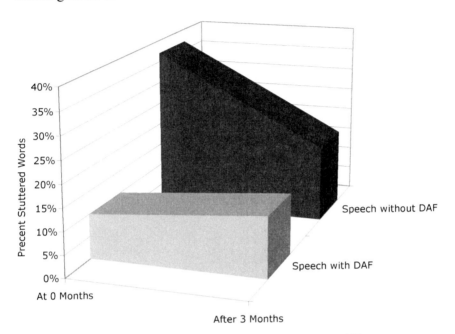

Figure 2: Long-Term Effects of DAF

The increase (from 10% to 13%) in stuttering when wearing the devices wasn't statistically significant. Examining this more closely, stuttering when wearing the device increased only for "automatic speech," such as reciting days of the week, and for repeating words and sentences after the examiner. No change in effectiveness was found in conversations or in a "picture description" task. This suggests that any "wearing off" effects occurred in less-important speaking situations.

The "carryover fluency" effect was the same across all speaking tasks.

In another study, an eleven-year-old boy received fourteen hours of structured therapy with mediated learning and a Casa Futura Technologies School DAF. His stuttering diminished from 9% dysfluencies to 5% dysfluencies (when speaking without the device, a 47% improvement). One year later he still had 5% dysfluencies. Another fourteen hours of treatment reduced his stuttering to 4% dysfluencies.[22]

Two other studies combined speech therapy with a DAF device. One study was of adults,[23] the other of children.[24] Both studies found that combining DAF and stuttering therapy trained the subjects to speak fluently (less than 2% stuttering) and no longer need the devices.

Frequency-Shifted Auditory Feedback

Frequency-shifted auditory feedback (FAF) shifts the pitch of your voice in your earphones. A FAF *upshift* makes you hear your voice sounding like Mickey Mouse. A FAF *downshift* makes you hear your voice sounding like a gravel-voiced radio announcer saying his station's call letters.

A quarter-octave pitch shift reduces stuttering about 35%. A half-octave pitch shift reduces stuttering about 65-70%. A full-octave pitch shift reduces stuttering about 70-75%. Combining DAF and FAF reduces stuttering about 80%.

Shifting pitch up or down is equally effective in short-term studies. But there may be long-term differences between up- and downshifts. FAF causes non-stutterers to speak at a higher or lower vocal pitch, depending on whether the device is set for an up or down frequency shift.[25] This higher or lower pitch vocal pitch results from changing vocal fold tension. In other words, FAF induces changes in vocal fold tension in non-stutterers.

A study found that my company's FAF devices, set for a half-octave downshift, didn't cause a change in vocal pitch in stutterers.[26] But speech clinics have reported that my FAF devices induce vocal fold relaxation in stutterers. Usually, stutterers need a greater pitch shift, between one-half and one octave down. Also, the study used older headphones which lacked the bass response of today's headphones. A new study might find that current devices, set to one-half or one octave down, induce vocal fold relaxation.

I've also seen FAF downshifts induce a slower speaking rate, similar to DAF. If this effect is consistent, then a FAF downshift should produce long-term carryover fluency.

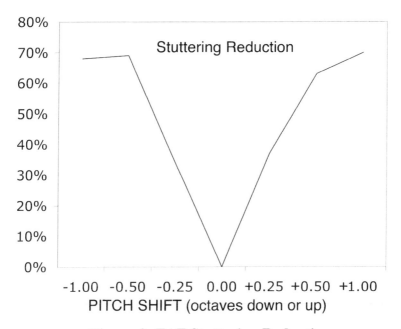

Figure 3: FAF Stuttering Reduction

Conversely, a FAF upshift (the Mickey Mouse voice) appears to induce vocal fold tension. I've seen FAF upshifts induce faster speaking rates. If this effect is consistent, then a FAF upshift should result in poor long-term performance (e.g., no carryover fluency, and possibly "wearing off").

Types of FAF

All published studies of FAF used *octave-scale* FAF. Octave-scale FAF requires lots of computing power (a *fast Fourier transformation*). My company's devices use octave-scale FAF. When you set my devices to a one-octave upshift, the 125-Hz fundamental frequency of an adult male voice is shifted up to 250 Hz. The 250 Hz first overtone of your voice is shifted to 500 Hz. The 500 Hz second overtone of your voice is shifted to 1000 Hz. And so on.

If you instead use a one-octave downshift, your 125 Hz voice is shifted in your earphones to 62 Hz. Your 250 Hz first overtone is shifted to 125 Hz, and so on.

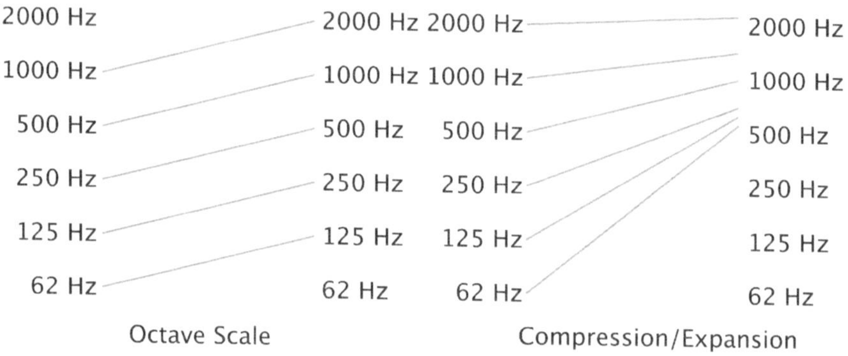

2000 Hz	2000 Hz	2000 Hz	2000 Hz
1000 Hz	1000 Hz	1000 Hz	1000 Hz
500 Hz	500 Hz	500 Hz	500 Hz
250 Hz	250 Hz	250 Hz	250 Hz
125 Hz	125 Hz	125 Hz	125 Hz
62 Hz	62 Hz	62 Hz	62 Hz
Octave Scale		Compression/Expansion	

Figure 4: Octave-Scale vs. Frequency-Compression FAF

But some devices made by other companies don't have enough processing power to produce octave-scale FAF. Instead, a simpler process uses frequency compression/expansion FAF. This sounds like the *ring modulators* used to make robot and alien voices in old science fiction movies. The upshift adds 500 Hz to your voice (or 1000 Hz or 2000 Hz, depending on the setting). Thus, your 125 Hz fundamental frequency is shifted to 625 Hz—more than two octaves up! Your 250 Hz first overtone is shifted to 750 Hz. Your 500 Hz second overtone is shifted to 1000 Hz.

When you downshift or *subtract* 500 Hz from your voice, your 125 Hz fundamental frequency vanishes. 125 Hz minus 500 Hz is nothing (there are no negative frequencies). The 250 Hz first overtone of your voice also vanishes. And the 500 Hz second overtone of your voice vanishes. You can only hear the weak third (1000 Hz) and higher overtones of your voice. When I tried another company's anti-stuttering device, I heard my voice in my ear *rise* in pitch as the FAF was adjusted lower!

No published studies have investigated whether frequency compression/expansion FAF has an effect on stuttering. A speech-language pathologist who works with such devices reported that frequency expansion (downshifting) "does not enhance fluency."[27]

Long-Term Effects of DAF Combined with FAF

Nine stutterers used a DAF/FAF device about seven hours per day, for twelve months.[28] The delay was set at 60 milliseconds and the frequency compression FAF at 500 Hz up. The subjects received brief speech therapy, specifically to prolong vowels and use "starter sounds" such as "um" and "ah."

At the start of the study, the DAF/FAF device reduced stuttering about 85%. Twelve months later, the subjects experienced no statistically significant "wearing off" of the devices' effectiveness. The subjects' speech without the devices didn't improve.

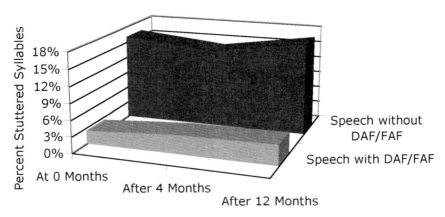

Figure 5: Long-term effectiveness of DAF/FAF device

Another study of the same type of device raised questions of whether long-term use could make stutterers' speech *worse*. Of six stutterers who used the device 10–23 months, two had speech about the same and four had speech much worse than before using the device. On average, stuttering increased about 50% after 18 months.[29]

Why did one anti-stuttering device produce 55% carryover fluency (page 16), when another anti-stuttering device produced no carryover, or possibly made the subjects' speech worse? Speculatively, upward FAF has positive immediate effects but negative long-term effects. Hearing your voice shifted up may improve your auditory processing but make your speech motor activity worse (i.e., make you speak with tighter vocal folds). If the auditory processing effect goes away when the device is removed, but the speech motor changes are retained, then no carryover would result.

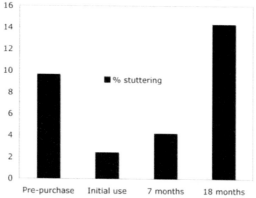

Figure 6: Long-term effectiveness of a DAF/FAF device

Or possibly the subjects using anti-stuttering devices for thirty minutes of practice per day slowed down their speech, improving their fluent speech motor skills; while subjects wearing anti-stuttering devices all day spoke at normal speaking rates, possibly making their auditory processing worse (page 15).

Masking Auditory Feedback (MAF)

If you have silent blocks, in which you can't make a sound, you'll want a device with masking auditory feedback (MAF). You push a button and the device pulls you out of the block.

MAF is a synthesized sine wave at your fundamental frequency (not "white noise"). This sound fools your brain into thinking that your vocal folds are vibrating. Your vocal folds relax and start vibrating.

The Edinburgh Masker, popular in the 1980s, helped many stutterers improve their speech over time, until they no longer needed the device. Other stutterers found that the device "wore off" and became ineffective. Still other stutterers have used the device for more than twenty years with no carryover or "wearing off." No research investigated why the device had different effects on different people. My guess is that some users used the devices to support therapy skills, but others used the devices to avoid therapy and support poor motor skills.

Sound Quality

A study found that a DAF/FAF anti-stuttering device made by my company was more than twice as effective as a DAF/FAF device made by another company.[30] The difference in effectiveness may have been due to differences in sound quality, e.g., listening to Beethoven played by a symphony orchestra isn't the same as hearing Beethoven as a cellphone ringtone.

Frequency Range

Different anti-stuttering devices have different frequency ranges. Generally, the bigger the microphone and earphones, the wider the frequency range.

My company's devices have a flat frequency response from 60 to 5000 Hz. This is the human vocal range, plus additional low range for FAF downshifting.

In contrast, hearing aids typically have a frequency range of 200 to 7000 Hz. The frequency ranges typically aren't flat, but instead are tuned to sound best somewhere between 3000 and 4000 Hz[31] (where most people lose their hearing). Hearing aids can't reproduce the low range of human voices, especially the fundamental frequency of phonation that's key to stuttering therapy.

Monaural vs. Binaural Sound

Binaural (two ears) sound is 25% more effective than monaural (one ear) sound.[32] My company's devices can be used either binaurally or monaurally. Other devices are monaural only.

Background Noise

Some anti-stuttering devices work well in quiet speech clinics, but are unusable in a noisy classroom or restaurant.

Noise-Canceling Microphones

Positioned correctly, a *noise-canceling directional microphone* eliminates background noise at the source. In contrast, the *omnidirectional microphones* in hearing aids, lapel microphones, and the smaller cellphone earsets pick up background noises louder than your voice.

Push-To-Talk Button

A "push to talk" button also eliminates background noise. You push a button and the device switches sound on. You let go of the button and the sound switches off.

In noisy environments you're usually in a group. For example, you go out to a restaurant with three friends. You talk one-fourth of the time. Most of the time you sit and listen, with clear hearing. When you have something to say, you push the button.

A push-to-talk button also works well for a child in school, who mostly listens and occasionally is called on by the teacher.

High-Frequency Filters

Most anti-stuttering devices have high-frequency filters to reduce noise above your vocal range.

Voice Activation

Voice activation switches on sound when the user talks, and switches off sound when the user stops talking. Voice activation works well if the device has a noise-canceling directional microphone. If the device has an omnidirectional microphone, loud noises switch on sound.

My company's Pocket Speech Lab analyzes your vocal fold tension and switches on DAF/FAF when you tense your vocal folds, before you stutter. It switches off sound when you're speaking with relaxed vocal folds, or not talking.

Dynamic Expansion

Some devices have dynamic expansion. This makes loud sounds

louder and quiet sounds quieter. If you're using a noise-canceling directional microphone this makes your voice louder and background sounds quieter. With an omnidirectional microphone it can make your voice quieter and background noise louder.

Acoustical Transparency
Listening to someone talk, while you wear a DAF device that's picking up the other person's voice, is like reading the following:

difficult to hear another person speaking

That says, "difficult to hear another person speaking." You hear the person speaking twice, with the words out of sync.

In contrast, quarter-octave FAF pitch shifts have little impact on your hearing.[33] It's like hearing a tune played simultaneously on a violin and on a viola. This is called "acoustically transparent."

Hearing Safety

Some anti-stuttering devices occlude (block) the ear that the device is in. Some anti-stuttering devices pick up, distort, and amplify background noise. Either results in temporary hearing impairment while wearing the device. If a child can't hear his teacher, he'll fall behind in school. Or he might get hit by a bus that he didn't hear coming.

Permanent hearing damage is also a concern. Underwriters Laboratories tested one of my company's anti-stuttering devices and found that the maximum volume couldn't cause hearing damage. But regardless of what lab tests found, have your hearing tested before buying an anti-stuttering device. If you experience ringing in your ears or pain from loud noises (e.g., a siren going by), discontinue using the device and get your hearing re-tested.

Should Children Use Anti-Stuttering Devices?
Children under six shouldn't use anti-stuttering devices. Preschool

stuttering therapy is usually 100% effective, so anti-stuttering devices are unnecessary.

Six- to thirteen-year-olds can use anti-stuttering devices under the supervision of a speech-language pathologist or a parent trained by a speech-language pathologist, or for *limited* unsupervised uses such as a classroom presentation. If your child gets speech therapy in school only twenty minutes each week, buying a device can enable your child to do therapy at home for thirty minutes every day, e.g., ten minutes reading aloud, a ten-minute conversation with a family member, and a ten-minute telephone call (perhaps to a grandparent).

We don't know whether children who stutter have the same neurological abnormalities that adult stutterers have. Altering a child's brain activity might cause his brain to develop in a different way. Extensive use of an anti-stuttering device might cause the child's brain to develop normal auditory processing and the child to outgrow stuttering. But perhaps extensive use of an anti-stuttering device would cause the child's brain to develop in another, unknown abnormal way. Until we know more about the brains of children who stutter, I suggest that children only use anti-stuttering devices if they want to, and the parents clearly hear improved fluency with on-target speech motor skills (e.g., relaxed vocal folds) when using the device.

Third-Party Payment

Most Americans who stutter can get anti-stuttering devices free.

Many states have *special telephone equipment distribution programs* that provide telephone-compatible anti-stuttering devices free to qualified residents. Some programs have income restrictions. These states include Arizona, California, Georgia, Maryland, Massachusetts, Missouri, North Carolina, Pennsylvania, Texas, and Wisconsin.

If you're unemployed, your state's *vocational rehabilitation* program will help you get a job, including paying for speech therapy and/or an anti-stuttering device.

In every case we know of, when a stutterer asked his or her *employer* for assistance paying for one of our devices, the employer was more than happy to help. Often the employer then offers the stutterer a promotion.

Many of our devices are paid for by *health insurance*. Speech clinics handle this billing. Casa Futura Technologies never directly bills health insurance plans.

We've had good experiences with *service organizations* including Sertoma (SERvice TO MAnkind) and Lions Clubs. Our experience has been that service organizations prefer to help low-income children and teenagers, and that they prefer to be approached by the child's speech-language pathologist.

We've also had devices paid for by Veterans Administration Medical Centers and Medicaid.

I'm not an expert on how foreign countries pay for health care. (In fact, I'm completely bewildered!)

For more about these and other programs, see my website

http://www.casafuturatech.com/Catalog/discounts.shtml

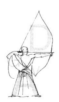

Fluency Shaping Therapy

Watch a stutterer struggle to talk. You see that stuttering is primarily overtense, overstimulated respiration, vocal folds, and articulation (lips, jaw, and tongue) muscles. Brain scans of adult stutterers have found overactivity in the left caudate nucleus speech motor (muscle) control area, during stuttering. This suggests there's a neurological basis for these overactive speech-production muscles.

Fluency shaping therapy treats this problem. It trains stutterers to speak with relaxed respiration, relaxed vocal folds, and relaxed articulation muscles.

This chapter is longer than any other chapter. Fluency shaping therapy is where you learn to talk fluently. If you don't master these skills, none of the other treatments—medications, anti-stuttering devices, handling stress better, and psychological interventions—will be fully effective.

Conversely, you may have tried fluency shaping therapy and it didn't work for you. What I call "fluency shaping therapy" is different from the fluency shaping therapy practiced at most speech clinics. I've added a theoretical basis for why fluency shaping therapy works (motor learning and control); new therapy skills (e.g., lower vocal pitch); and a chapter about making fluent speech automatic and effortless ("Beyond Fluency Shaping," page 57).

Motor Learning and Control

Motor learning and control is the study of how brains execute complex muscle movements. Physical therapy and occupational therapy students study motor learning and control. Speech pathology students don't (at least not for treating stuttering).

Sports coaches also study motor learning and control. The principles of motor learning and control are usually illustrated with examples from gymnastics, tennis, golf, or other sports.

Closed-Loop Motor Control

A muscle movement takes about 200 milliseconds (one-fifth of a second) to execute:

1. *Sensation*, or neural transmission from sensory receptors in your eyes, ears, etc., to your brain, takes about 15 milliseconds.

2. *Perception*, which retrieves long-term memories to organize, classify, and interpret your sensations, takes about 45 milliseconds. *Perception* changes *sensation* data into perceived information or meaning.

3. *Response selection* takes about 75 milliseconds. You use current perception and past experiences to formulate a course or action. For example, in baseball, a batter watches the pitcher and decides whether to swing at a pitch, hit or bunt, hit to left field or right, etc. Psychologists differentiate conscious *decisions* from unconscious translations, or relating a particular stimulus to a particular response.

4. *Response execution* of an action plan—a step-by-step sequence of events that make up the planned movement— takes about 15 milliseconds. In these events, motor neurons carry signals from the brain or spinal cord to muscles.

Under *closed-loop motor control* you use perception to consciously, continuously adjust muscle movements. For example, threading a needle. You look at the needle. You look at the thread. You move the thread towards the needle. You look at the needle again. You look at the thread again. You correct your movement. You do this dozens of times until the thread is through the needle.

Each *stimulus-response* adjustment takes at least 200 milliseconds (one-fifth of a second). If you make ten adjustments, the task takes at least two seconds.

Closed-loop motor control has two advantages. It enables precise control, and it enables execution of novel movements (activities you've never done before). For example, threading a needle on the deck of a rolling ship.

Closed-loop motor control has two disadvantages. It's slow, and it requires your full attention.

Closed-loop motor control is good for learning new skills, or for executing skills you rarely need. But you don't want to use closed-loop motor control for fast-paced, frequently used skills.

Open-Loop Motor Control
200 milliseconds—a split second—may seem fast, but it's too slow for many motor tasks. For example, a gymnast's double-back somersault requires muscle movements lasting only tens of milliseconds.

How is it possible to execute a muscle movement in tens of milliseconds, when the sensation to execution cycle requires about 200 milliseconds? Simple—don't do the sensation, perception, and response selection stages. Just do the response execution. This final stage of muscle movements can be performed in as little as 15 milliseconds. This is called *open-loop motor control*. Open-loop motor control is the execution of preprogrammed movements, called a *motor program*, without perceptual feedback.

The colloquial term for this is "muscle memory." For example, gymnasts practice hours each day for years, until their muscles seem to know what to do without the mind getting involved.

After winning the gold medal in gymnastics at the 1984 Olympics, Mary Lou Retton said that coach

Bela [Karolyi] can really teach, I've learned so much from him. Many long hours were spent in the gymnasium...repetition, feedback, repetition, and experimentation. Somehow, after a lot of bumps and bruises, it got easier, as if I could float.

Karolyi added,

> Someone should be able to sneak up and drag you out at midnight and push you out on some strange floor, and you should be able to do your entire routine sound asleep in your pajamas. Without a mistake. That's the secret. It's got to be a natural reaction.

Open-loop motor control has two advantages:

1. It's fast. You can execute muscle movements with split-second timing.
2. It requires no attention. Movements under open-loop control are *automatic* and mentally *effortless*.

Open-loop motor control has three disadvantages:

1. If your motor program contains errors, you'll execute the errors. You can't stop and adjust a mistake. You may not even be aware that you made a mistake.
2. Developing open-loop control of a motor skill requires long practice—especially for adults. Children learn some motor skills easily, that adults struggle for years to master.
3. Novel or new situations can't be handled. For example, in the 2000 Olympics, officials set the gymnastic vault two inches too low. The officials didn't correct the height until 18 of the 36 women had performed. These 18 athletes performed poorly, eliminating their hopes of winning medals. The American hopeful, Elise Ray, suffered a "devastating fall."[34]

Learning New Motor Skills

Use closed-loop motor control for learning a new motor skill. Then gradually increase your speed until you can perform the motor skill using open-loop motor control.

For example, if you take tennis or golf lessons the coach will have you start with swinging the club or racquet slowly. When you've perfected your form, your coach will have you gradually increase the speed and force, while maintaining form. After extensive practice you'll be executing perfect open-loop motor programs. You'll smash the ball hard and fast and accurately without paying attention to your elbows or knees or anything other than the ball.

Speech Motor Control

Normal speech uses open-loop motor control:

1. Speech is *fast*. Phonemes (speech sounds) are typically 20 to 40 milliseconds.
2. Speech is *complex*, requiring coordination of hundreds of muscles to produce sounds.
3. Speech is *automatic* and *effortless*. Speakers think about what they're saying, not about the muscles they're moving.

Fluency shaping stuttering therapy uses closed-loop speech motor control. You consciously relax your breathing. Then, as you exhale, you slowly increase your vocal fold tension, until your vocal folds hum. Then you slowly move your lips, jaw, and tongue to form the sounds of each word. Stuttering is impossible when using closed-loop speech motor control. Stuttering dysfluencies are open-loop speech motor programs.

Making stuttering impossible might sound appealing, but

1. Closed-loop speech motor control is slow. Closed-loop motor control takes about 200 milliseconds per muscle movement. Open-loop speech sounds are typically in the

20-40 millisecond range. Closed-loop speech motor control slows speech five to ten times, or one or two seconds per syllable.

2. Closed-loop speech motor control demands your full attention. You must pay attention to your breathing, vocal folds, and lips, jaw, and tongue. This isn't a problem when reading a list of words, but is difficult to use in conversations.

3. Your speech loses prosody (emotional intonation). You sound like a robot with dying batteries.

Prosody, Parameterization Schemata, and Response Selection

Why closed-loop speech motor control loses prosody is an interesting question.

A study of television talk show guests found that 94% of what viewers remembered was prosody, or what actors call *emoting*, or what lawyers call *affect*.[35] Much—or almost all—meaning is communicated by prosody. *Schemata theory* suggests that you learn certain *invariable characteristics* of a motor skill, and you learn certain execution rules or *parameterization schemata*. You then combine the invariable elements with the rules to produce a motor plan.

For example, in a public speaking class I once read algebra problems in an angry voice, in a sad voice, and then with the rhythm and emotional intonation of a stand-up comedian. The algebra problems were invariable—I read the same algebra problems each time. I changed the parameterization schemata to communicate different emotional states. Amazingly, the audience laughed at the "punchlines" when I did the stand-up comedy delivery. Even though the "punchlines" were just numbers, I made the audience think that a punchline was coming, and they laughed at the right times. 94% of the joke was the delivery.

Accents are another parameterization schema that conveys meaning. For example, a waitress from Oklahoma asked me if I wanted *ah-iss*. When I figured out that she was asking about ice, I affirmatively answered *yay-iss*. I knew the invariable characteristics of "yes," and when I'd learned the rules of an Oklahoma accent—e.g., break monosyllabic words into two syllables—I was able to say a word I'd never heard.

In normal speech, we produce *prosody* through unconscious *response selection* of *parameterization schemata*. Different environmental cues cause us to select different responses. For example, you walk into a church and immediately lower your vocal volume. But if no one else is in the church, you could yell "I hate to wear pants!" while turning somersaults down the aisle. OK, that's one of my eccentric hobbies, but most people wouldn't do that.

Another example is a person who grew up spending summers in Vermont and winters in Georgia. When she's in New England she speaks in a Yankee accent. When she's in the South she switches to a southern accent. Different environmental cues cause her to unconsciously select different parameterization schema to produce each accent.

Like prosody and accents, stuttering is a parameterization schema. A stutterer responds to environmental cues to unconsciously select fluent speech parameters or stuttering speech parameters, which are then combined with invariable characteristics of words to produce fluent or stuttered speech. Thus you can treat stuttering by training stutterers to respond differently to environmental cues ("Responding to Stress," page 76), or by training stutterers to use fluent speech parameterization schema (this chapter).

Training a stutterer to not feel fear or anxiety when answering the telephone is changing the response selection to an environmental cue (a ringing telephone). In contrast, training a stutterer to speak with relaxed vocal folds changes a speech parameter.

Snake Oil and Charlatans

Closed-loop speech motor control is the "wizard behind the curtain" of many stuttering therapy programs. Switch any stutterer to closed-loop speech motor control and he or she will be completely fluent.

You can switch to closed-loop speech motor control by making any speech process conscious instead of unconscious. For example, focusing on relaxed, slow breathing will switch you into closed-loop speech motor control, with your vocal folds and articulators (lips, jaw, and tongue) following right along. Or you can focus on producing "gentle onsets" with your vocal folds. This will switch your breathing and articulators to closed-loop speech motor control. Or you can focus on "reduced articulatory pressure" and your breathing and vocal folds will follow.

Always these "wizards" claim that their therapies are 100% effective if the stutterer "really tries," that is, if he devotes his full attention to closed-loop speech motor control. If he instead pays attention to a conversation, switches into open-loop speech motor control, and then stutters, then he wasn't "really trying."

And the closed-loop speech motor control effect has caused speech-language pathologists to hypothesize that stutterers have something wrong with their breathing, or with their vocal folds, or with their articulators, or even that stutterers' brains are slow in some way. That latter theory is like saying that student drivers have slower brains than Indy 500 race car drivers because student drivers are safe at 20 mph but crash when driving at 200 mph. Everyone performs slowly when attentively learning a new motor skill, then their speed improves with practice. For stutterers in speech therapy, the new motor skill is fluent speech.

Some speech clinics tell stutterers that they'll always have to speak slowly. That's like training a student driver to drive 20 mph, then telling him never to go faster.

Slow Speech Is Not the Goal of Stuttering Therapy
If you learn tennis or golf, you'll use closed-loop motor control when you're learning to swing the club or racquet. As you practice, increasing your speed and force, you'll gradually reinforce open-loop motor programs.

Similarly, you'll use closed-loop speech motor control when working with your speech-language pathologist. She'll train you to move your respiration muscles, vocal folds, and articulators correctly to produce fluent speech. When you've mastered this at a very slow speaking rate, she'll help you to gradually increase your speaking rate, while staying fluent. The goal is fluent, automatic, effortless, normal-sounding and normal-rate speech. Slow speech is not the goal of stuttering therapy.

Severe stutterers usually don't mind learning closed-loop speech motor control. If your stuttered speech is ten to twenty times slower than normal speech, then closed-loop speech motor control, which is typically five to ten times slower than normal speech, will double your speaking rate. Some severe stutterers are even willing to use closed-loop speech motor control outside of the speech clinic. Record conversations with and without using closed-loop speech motor control. Count your syllables per second. You may find that closed-loop speech motor control feels slower but is actually faster than your stuttered speech.

But mild stutterers don't like closed-loop speech motor control. They can hide their stuttering by avoidance and substitution (of certain sounds, words, or speaking situations). They can sound fluent at a normal speaking rate. Closed-loop speech motor control would "advertise to the world" that they have a speech disorder. If they're embarrassed to admit that they stutter, they won't want to use closed-loop speech motor control.

Mild stutterers should consider that closed-loop speech motor control enables them to say anything they want. For example, a mild stutterer wants to buy a chess set. He's afraid of *s* words, so he calls a toy store and asks if they have "one of those games with kings and knights and castles."

The puzzled clerk responds that the store has many games with kings and castles and knights. After five minutes of conversation, the clerk asks, "Do you mean *chess sets?*" The stutterer says yes. The clerk never knows that the caller is a stutterer, but she thinks that the caller is an idiot. The stutterer wasted five minutes because he wasn't willing to use ten seconds of slow speech.

Or the stutterer drives to the store and looks for a chess set, without calling first. If the store doesn't have chess sets he wastes an hour, to save ten seconds. Saying what you want slowly is faster than saying something else, or not speaking.

Analogy to Touchtyping

I've never taken a typing class. I type with two fingers, about 45 words per minute. (I'm probably the world's fastest two-fingered typist!)

I've tried to learn touchtyping. My speed dropped to less than ten words per minute. Touchtyping not only slowed me down, it required my full concentration. I couldn't think about what I was writing, only about moving my fingers.

I gave up touchtyping within a week. If I'd kept at it, my speed would have increased and eventually surpassed my two-fingered typing speed. I might have been typing 80 words per minute now. The mental effort would have diminished, until touchtyping was automatic and effortless.

Coaches say they'd rather work with a novice who has never played their sport, rather than with an experienced player who uses incorrect techniques. It's easier to learn a new motor skill correctly than it is to correct an incorrect, deeply ingrained motor skill.

Stuttering is difficult to overcome because we learned to talk incorrectly. We have to learn new, fluent speech motor skills, *and* we have to not use our old, dysfluent speech motor skills. We learned these dysfluent speech motor skills in childhood, when our brains were growing. Now the dysfluent speech motor skills are hardwired into our brains. Making fluent speech automatic and effortless, for a stutterer, demands more time and effort than learning a new sport or vocational skill.

Using DAF to Slow Speaking Rate

Many speech clinics use delayed auditory feedback (DAF) devices to establish fluency using closed-loop speech motor control. With only a little training a DAF device can help a stutterer maintain perfectly paced, steady, mentally effortless, slow closed-loop speech motor control.

The user's speaking rate can adjusted by turning a knob. A typical protocol is to train a stutterer to use closed-loop speech motor control with a 200-millisecond delay and one to two seconds per syllable. The stutterer practices this until he is 100% fluent. That usually takes only one or two therapy sessions. (A study found that without training a 195-millisecond delay reduced stuttering only 85%.[36])

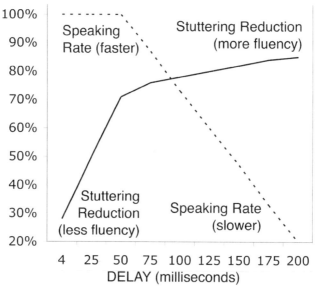

Figure 7: DAF Effectiveness and Speaking Rate

When the stutterer can speak 100% fluently, the speech-language pathologist then has the stutterer use one- or two-second stretched syllables without the DAF device; in increasingly stressful situations (e.g., calling the speech-language pathologist's answering machine); and then with the DAF device adjusted for faster speaking rates. The stutterer must stay on-target with 100% fluency, or go back to using the DAF device at 200 milliseconds and a one- to two-second speaking rate.

Typically, a 100-millisecond DAF delay is used with half-second per syllable stretched speech, a 75-millisecond delay is used with quarter-second per syllable "slow normal" speech, and a 50-millisecond delay is used with a normal speaking rate.

Three Stages of Motor Learning

We learn new muscle movements, or *motor skills*, in three stages:

1. In the *cognitive stage*, an instructor demonstrates the motor skill to you.
2. In the *associative stage*, you learn to perform and refine the motor skill. You perform the movements under closed-loop control.
3. In the *autonomous stage*, the motor skill becomes automatic. You perform the muscle movements without mental effort. You perform the movements under open-loop control.

For example, imagine yourself learning to play golf or tennis. You watch the coach hit a few practice balls. Then the coach hands you the club or racket. The coach guides you through a swing, telling you to drop this shoulder or extend that forearm. Soon you can execute the swing perfectly, if you fully concentrate on each movement. You then practice the swing, and your game improves.

A few years later a novice admires your excellent swing and asks you to explain how you do it. "I don't know," you say, "I just do it without thinking about it."

For another example, last summer I tried mountain bike racing. In four races I crashed four times. I then hired a coach. In twelve hours over three weeks, he taught me how to ride down hills, make tight turns, jump my bike over logs, climb hills, plus a few tricks such as picking up a water bottle off the ground.

Then I quit mountain bike racing. I'd completed the associative stage and learned how to do each skill. Now I would have to practice these skills hours a day, several times a week for years to make the skills automatic in the fast, high-stress environment of racing. In other words, I could do any of the skills if I thought about it, but my body didn't automatically execute the moves without conscious mental effort. I decided that mountain bike racing isn't important enough to me to spend thousands of hours practicing skills.

Stuttering therapy follows a similar course. A speech-language pathologist can show you the fluency skills—relaxed, diaphragmatic breathing; vocal fold relaxation (gentle onsets); and relaxed articulation muscles (lips, jaw, and tongue)—in ten minutes. Teaching you to execute these skills takes a few hours. You can then speak fluently in the speech clinic, when you mentally concentrate on each skill. Almost everyone successfully completes these cognitive and associative stages.

You then have to practice these skills thousands of hours to make them automatic and effortless, in high-stress situations. Many stutterers fail at this stage. But no one intentionally fails for the reasons I quit mountain bike racing. No one rationally weighs the alternatives and says, "Talking isn't important to me. I'll learn sign language instead, or write notes."

Instead, stutterers fail at the autonomous stage because speech clinics don't train this well. Speech clinics call this *transfer*. Perhaps your speech-language pathologist takes you to a shopping mall for a few hours. But the autonomous stage requires thousands of hours of conversations, including high-stress conversations. Stutterers habitually avoid such conversations. You may find that the skills you learned in the low-stress speech clinic fail in high-stress conversations. Your therapy progress begins to fail. You revert to old habits and avoidances. Your stuttering returns.

The next chapter will detail the autonomous stage. The rest of this chapter presents what you learn in the cognitive and associative stages.

Fluency-Shaping Techniques

Fluency shaping therapy programs typically begin with slow speech with stretched vowels, then work on relaxed, diaphragmatic breathing, then work on vocal fold awareness and control, and finally work on relaxed articulation (lips, jaw, and tongue).

These techniques are all abnormal. They all produce "weird"-sounding speech. The idea is to go to extremes when practicing (in the speech clinic or at home), and then in "real world" conversations you reduce the techniques so that you sound normal, and speak fluently.

Choosing a Speech-Language Pathologist

Find a speech-language pathologist who specializes in stuttering. About 100,000 speech-language pathologists are licensed by the American Speech-Language Hearing Association (ASHA). Of these, fewer than 400 are board-certified Fluency Specialists. These specialists are listed on the website

http://www.stutteringspecialists.org/

The Stuttering Foundation of America also lists speech-language pathologists. This webpage is

http://www.stuttersfa.org/referral.htm

You could also go to a National Stuttering Association local support group and ask for recommendations. Their website is

http://www.nsastutter.org/

Is Self-Therapy an Option?

You can't learn motor skills out of a book. You can learn the *cognitive* stage from a book or video. Analogously, many video-tapes offer to teach golfers how to improve their swing.

But the *associative* stage requires *feedback*. A trained individual must observe you and tell you when your performance is correct, when your performance is incorrect, and what to change to correct your performance.

This book comes with a DVD ("Anti-Stuttering Devices Demo and Training") demonstrating two fluency skills: slow speech with stretched vowels, and lower vocal pitch with relaxed breathing and relaxed vocal folds. The video can also be downloaded from my website (http://www.casafutura.com). If it helps you, great. If not, make an appointment at a speech clinic.

Slow Speech with Stretched Vowels

Let's start with how not to do slow speech with stretched vowels:

"I" < pause> "am" < pause> "an" < pause> "American."

Saying "I am an American" normally takes about 1.5 seconds (seven syllables at about five syllables per second). By silently pausing two seconds between words, and saying each word normally, the phrase would take about eight seconds. That would not improve your fluency.

Instead, stretch each vowel for a second or two. Also stretch voiced consonants (e.g., /m/, /n/, /r/) a little longer then normal, but not as long as vowels. Articulate voiceless consonants (e.g., /k/) lightly and quickly, just touching your lips or tongue and then moving to the next voiced sound.

Join the syllables together, with no breaks or pauses between words. The result should sound like:

"IIIIIIIaaaaammmaaaaannAAAAAmmeeeeerriiiiiiiikaaaaann"

Be sure that each syllable is held equally. In other words, "American" should take four times longer to say than "I." Don't make "American" the same length as "I."

Should you hold each syllable for one second or for two seconds? Some speech clinics start with one-second stretched syllables, when other speech clinics start with two seconds per syllable. No research has investigated which is more effective. If you are 100% fluent at one second per syllable, then that should be slow enough. But if you're not 100% fluent at one second per syllable, use two seconds per syllable. According to motor learning theory, you need to execute slow enough that your form is perfect, but there's no reason to execute slower.

Use a stopwatch to check that each syllable is the same length.

If you have a DAF device, set the delay to 200 milliseconds. Then hold each syllable until you hear yourself in the headphones. Check your stopwatch and you should see that each syllable is between one and two seconds.

Relaxed Breathing

Place one hand on your stomach. Breathe so that your hand moves out when you inhale, and in when you exhale.

Notice that you're taking many small breaths. Your inhale and exhale times are equal.

This is relaxed or *diaphragmatic* breathing. This is the way people normally breathe.

Now switch to upper-chest breathing or *thoracic* breathing. Take a big breath, using your upper chest muscles to expand your lungs. Release the air slowly, while maintaining this upper chest muscle tension to hold air in your lungs as long as possible. When you've released the air, quickly take another breath, filling your lungs as rapidly as possible.

Practice switching between thoracic and diaphragmatic breathing.

Thoracic breathing increases our lung capacity. It enables us to maximize our physical exertion. Our "fight or flight" instinct switches us to thoracic breathing. We're then better able to run or fight.

Some individuals *hyperventilate* or switch to thoracic breathing when experiencing non-physical stress. Stress reduction classes teach students to relax by switching to diaphragmatic breathing.

We also use thoracic breathing when talking. A large breath with a long, slow exhale enable us to speak many words before pausing for another breath.

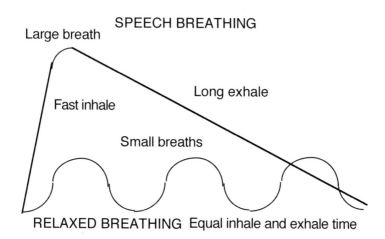

Figure 8: Thoracic vs. Diaphragmatic Breathing

Well-meaning people who know nothing about stuttering may tell you to "take a deep breath" before talking. But the opposite is better advice. Diaphragmatic breathing is the foundation of many stuttering therapy programs. Taking smaller breaths with your diaphragm can help you relax and talk fluently.

Try it. Your relaxed breathing will relax your entire body. Most importantly, it will relax your vocal folds, and then your lips, jaw, and tongue. Your voice will deepen and sound confident and even "sexy." You'll feel relaxed and confident.

Practice a word list (page 175) using diaphragmatic breathing. Read a magazine page aloud using diaphragmatic breathing.

You'll soon discover a few problems trying to speak with diaphragmatic breathing. Each breath is small, so you're able to say only a few words on each breath. Inhale time and exhale time are equal, so you have long pauses between short phrases. You're unable to speak loudly.

Like other fluent speech motor skills, speaking with diaphragmatic breathing is abnormal but useful. Include speaking with diaphragmatic breathing in your stuttering therapy practice exercises. Mastering this skill will enable you to speak short phrases fluently in stressful situations. For example, a police officer pulls you over for speeding. You don't need to say much besides, "Yes, officer," and "No, officer."

And as you master speaking with diaphragmatic breathing, you'll develop something in-between thoracic and diaphragmatic breathing. This "in-between" breathing will be more relaxed than thoracic breathing, yet your phrase length and vocal volume will be within the normal range.

Phonation

Your vocal folds are flaps of muscle in your throat. Making your vocal folds vibrate produces sound. This sound then becomes your voice. Vocal fold vibration is called *phonation.*

Two conditions produce phonation. First, you release air from your lungs. Next, you tension or tighten your vocal folds.

Place your fingers on your throat. Exhale and hum. Your fingers should feel a vibration. This is your vocal folds vibrating.

Stop humming, and feel the vibration stop. Practice switching your phonation on and off.

Now vary your phonation in two ways. Change your volume (hum louder, then quieter). Change your pitch. Hum up and down a musical scale.

How did you do that? You varied your volume of exhalation, i.e., you increased or decreased the air releasing from your lungs by tensing or relaxing your thoracic (upper chest) muscles. More exhalation enabled you to produce more volume.

You also varied your vocal fold tension. Tense vocal folds produce a higher-pitched voice. Relaxed vocal folds produce a deeper or lower-pitched voice.

Tense your vocal folds as hard as you can. You'll completely block your throat, not allowing any air to escape. If you take a deep breath and then block your throat, your increased lung pressure makes your chest stronger. Like inflating a tire to carry a heavier load, this is effective for lifting a heavy weight. But it's not a good way to talk!

Practice one more aspect of phonation. Take a breath and hold it, tense your vocal folds, then release air. Switch to the other way: take a breath, release a little air, then tense your vocal folds. Note that the former produced a croak. The latter produced a nice hum. This shows that phonation requires timing two muscle movements: exhaling a little air, and then starting to tense your vocal folds.

You now see that three things can go wrong with phonation:

1. Releasing too much or too little air (*inadequate breath support*).
2. Overtensing your vocal folds. Under stress, you may try too hard to talk, tense your vocal folds too much, and block off air flow. This results in a *silent block*.
3. Mistiming exhalation and vocal fold tension. A goal of stuttering therapy is train the stutterer to consciously take a breath, release a little air, gently tense his vocal folds, and then begin to talk. This exercise is called *gentle onset* or *easy onset*.

Gentle Onsets with Vowels

To hit a baseball home run, you use all of your arm muscle strength. In contrast, to putt a golf ball a few feet, your arm muscles are more relaxed than tense. Phonation is like putting a golf ball, not like hitting a home run.

To use *gentle onsets* (also called *easy onsets*), take a relaxed breath with your diaphragm. Release a little air. Make an *ah* sound as you gradually increase your vocal fold tension. Feel your vocal folds begin to vibrate. Increase your vocal fold tension, until you reach normal speaking volume. Gradually reduce vocal fold tension, until you reach silence. Time this to take about two seconds. You should be able to do this on one breath, without reaching residual air.

You can buy computer applications that display your phonation contour on the screen. Applications include Dr. Fluency, Speak:Gentle, and the Computer-Aided Fluency Establishment and Trainer (CAFET). Or you can use a sound-recording and -editing application (many such applications are available free). On a computer monitor, your vocal volume should look like this:

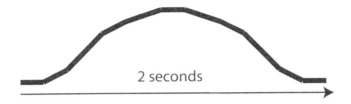

2 seconds

Figure 9: Gentle Onset Voice Contour

Practice fifteen gentle onsets with the fifteen vowel sounds (say the vowel, not the word):

Front Vowels:	long *e*, as in *beet*
	short *i*, as in *bit*
	long *a*, as in *bait*
	short *e*, as in *bet*
	short *a*, as in *at*
Back Vowels:	long *u*, as in *boot*
	short *o*, as in *book*
	long *o*, as in *boat*
	aw, as in *cause*
	ah, as in *cot*
Central Vowels:	*ow*, as in *about*
	short *u*, as in *but*
Dipthongs:	long *i*, as in *bite*
	oy, as in *boy*
	au, as in *bough*

Gentle Onsets with Words

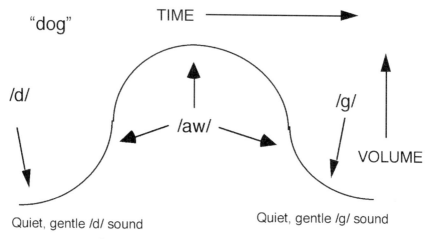

Quiet, gentle /d/ sound

Quiet, gentle /g/ sound

Stretched vowel /aw/ sound, begin
quietly, gently increase volume

Figure 10: Gentle Onset with Words

Now say "dog," stretched over two seconds, with gentle onset. Begin with a quiet, gentle /d/ sound. Switch to the /aw/ vowel sound and gradually increase vocal volume. After one second, gradually reduce vocal volume. Switch to the /g/ sound, and stop vocal fold vibration.

Voice and Voiceless Consonants

All vowels use phonation. Some consonants use phonation, i.e., are *voiced*. Other consonants are produced without phonation, i.e., are *voiceless*. You can whisper these consonants.

Place your fingers on your throat. Say *ah* to feel your vocal folds vibrating. Say the following words and decide whether the initial consonant is voice or voiceless:

/h/	hail	/w/	whale
/f/	famous	/v/	vacant
/s/	saber	/z/	zany
/sh/	chenille	/zh/	jeté (a ballet move)
/ch/	chive	/j/	jive

/thr/	throw	/th/	those
/p/	pipeline	/b/	bison
/t/	tie-dye	/d/	diner
/k/	kindness	/g/	guide

The first column was voiceless. The second column was voiced.

Did you notice that these sounds were pairs? /h/ and /w/ have your lips, jaw, and tongue in the same positions. The difference is that your vocal folds vibrate to produce /w/, but don't vibrate to produce /h/.

To say a word with a voiceless consonant, take a breath, let out a little air, shape the consonant with your lips, jaw, and tongue, then switch to the vowel and gently start your vocal fold vibration.

Practice a word list (page 175). Keep your fingers on your throat to feel your vocal folds switching on and off as you go from voiced to voiceless sounds. Stretch each word to two seconds.

Because most words contain both voiced and voiceless sounds, we switch our vocal folds on and off many times each second while talking. A core behavior of stuttering is an inability to switch phonation on at the right moments. The timing can be as precise as one one-hundredth (1/100) of a second.

Normal speech is about five syllables per second, or 0.2 seconds per syllable. For this practice you're using two seconds per syllable stretched speech, or ten times slower than a normal speaking rate. Slowing down your speech helps you develop awareness and control of speech elements that are otherwise too fast to notice or control. If you play a sport, such as tennis or golf, your coach might videotape your swing and then replay it back in slow motion. This improves your awareness and control of the motor skill.

Continuous Phonation

Stuttering therapy sometimes teaches techniques that produce fluency, but sound abnormal. For example, speech with diaphragmatic breathing produces fluency, but shortens phrase length and makes you pause between phrases. The immediate goal is to use these techniques to produce fluent speech, and over time reduce the degree of exaggeration, until your speech sounds normal. Another goal is have a "trick" to use in stressful situations, such as speaking to a police officer.

Continuous phonation is such a technique or trick. Recall that consonants come in voiced/voiceless pairs. Simple substitute a voiced consonant whenever you need to say a voiceless consonant.

For example, "Patty" becomes "Baddy." Say each word slowly, with your fingers on your throat to feel your phonation. You'll feel your vocal folds switch on and off for "Patty," but stay on for "Baddy."

If you shorten the consonants and stretch your vowels (producing a slower speaking rate), listeners won't hear the difference between "Patty" and "Baddy."

Gentle Onsets with Multisyllabic Words

Practice using a gentle onset on each syllable. Go loud on each vowel. On the consonants, relax, go quiet, and lightly and quickly articulate the sounds.

For example, on "American," you start with a gentle onset on the initial /uh/. Open your mouth wide at the loudest point in the phonation contour.

Take the /uh/ sound down in volume, while at the same time closing your mouth to articulate the voiced /m/. Bring the /eh/ sound up in volume. Again, open your mouth wide at the loudest point in the phonation contour.

Take the /eh/ sound down in volume, while at the same time reduce your jaw opening (but don't close your lips) to articulate the voiced /r/.

Open your mouth wide again for the /ih/ vowel on the third syllable.

Now you get to the only voiceless sound in "American." Before the /k/ sound, take the down the volume of the /ih/ vowel. Whisper the /k/. If you block, you dropped the /ih/ volume too fast. Try again with a long, slow decline in volume on the /ih/. Articulate the

/k/ lightly, for just a moment.

If you still block on the /k/, change it to a voiced /g/. In other words, say "Amerigan."

Use another gentle onset on the final /eh/ vowel. Reduce your volume on the final voiced /n/ consonant.

The result is an abnormal-sounding "sing-song" speech pattern. Your jaw opens and closes noticeably on each syllable. While you won't want to talk like this for the rest of your life, for practice or in stressful situations this technique helps you use gentle onsets, continuous phonation, and a slower speaking rate.

Articulation

The third set of speech muscles (after respiration and phonation) are your articulators: lips, jaw, and tongue. These muscles form your vocal fold humming into sounds and words. If you phonate without moving your lips, jaw, and tongue, all that comes out of your mouth is humming. The goal of this last target is to relax these muscles.

Reduced articulatory pressure is also called "soft targets."

Lightly touch your tongue for the /t/. Lightly close your lips for the /b/. Keep your speech production muscles relaxed for all sounds.

The wrong way is to tense your lips and tongue and jaw too much, and hold this tension too long.

You've learned to stretch and emphasize vowels. Now work on de-emphasizing consonants. If you stretch and emphasize vowels, and de-emphasize consonants, you should be able to speak fluently.

Read another word list (page 175) aloud. Feel how your lips, jaw, and tongue move to change sounds. Say each word with normal articulation tension. Then say the word again with tense articulation. Then say the word again with relaxed articulation.

Some stuttering therapy programs at this point devote many hours to teaching the stutterer the correct lips, jaw, and tongue position for each of the 40+ sounds of English. This is unnecessary, in my opinion. Stuttering is not an articulation disorder. Stutterers don't, in general, misarticulate sounds (e.g., saying /w/ instead of /v/). Stutterers instead need to learn to relax their lips, jaws, and tongues.

There are exceptions. If your speech-language pathologist diagnoses that you have articulation problems, or if you speak with a foreign accent, do articulation therapy to train you to place your lips, jaw, and tongue in the correct positions.

Computers and Electronics for Fluency Shaping

The associative stage of motor learning requires feedback. In sports this is called *knowledge of results*. For example, in golf or tennis you see where the ball goes after you hit it. Playing golf or tennis on a dark, foggy night would be impossible.

Feedback quality is affected by *speed*. If you hit ten golf balls on a dark, foggy night, then the next day find one of the balls 150 yards away, you'll have no memory of what you did right to hit it so far.

Feedback quality is also affected by *accuracy*. If you and your buddy each hit a golf ball, and one ball goes 150 yards but you don't know whose ball it was, you have inaccurate feedback.

Or the observer gets bored. If you hit golf balls for hours, and have a person telling you how far the balls go, sooner or later the person will stop paying attention.

Which Fluency Skills Need Feedback?
When you're learning fluent speech motor skills, you need knowledge of results. Some skills are easy to observe. For example, resting your hand on your stomach tells you whether you're using diaphragmatic (relaxed) breathing or thoracic (speech) breathing.

Your articulators (lips, jaw, and tongue) are a little harder to be aware of, as you can't see them. But you have good proprioceptive awareness of these muscles, so developing awareness and control isn't hard.

Your vocal folds are another story. These muscles are deep in your throat. You can't touch them or see them. Most people don't even know they have vocal folds.

The most difficult feedback is with the timing of all this. For example, your speech-language pathologist tells you to exhale a little air and then increase your vocal fold tension. You do this slowly and correctly. Then she tells you to increase the speed. You must execute these movements within hundredths of a second. You can't tell whether you're doing it right, and most speech-language pathologists can't either. A fluency specialist who's helped hundreds of stutterers has better-trained ear and visual skills and gives better quality of feedback than a speech-language pathologist who's never treated a stutterer.

Biofeedback Devices

Biofeedback is the measurement and display (to the user) of a physiological activity, to enable the user to improve awareness and control of the activity. Biofeedback machines provide:

1. Faster, more precise, and more reliable feedback than a human observer.
2. Machines can provide feedback in real-time, beeping the instant you make a mistake.
3. Machines can accurately measure things humans can't see or hear.
4. Machines never get bored, even after hours of practice.
5. With a computer training physical speech motor skills, a speech pathologist can spend more time on psychological aspects of stuttering.
6. If you learn visually rather than aurally, you may learn faster with a computer display than by listening to your speech on a tape recorder.
7. Some devices are designed for home practice use as well as clinical use.

But you still need a speech-language pathologist to train you to do the target motor skills (cognitive stage). The machines can only help you to refine your skills (associative stage).

CAFET and Dr. Fluency

The Computer-Aided Fluency Establishment and Trainer (CAFET) and Dr. Fluency are computer-based biofeedback systems. Both use a microphone to monitor vocal volume, as a surrogate for vocal fold activity, and a chest strap to monitor breathing.

You see your breathing and vocal volume displayed on the computer screen, along with instructions or error messages. The two computer systems train similar speech motor skills:

1. Relaxed, diaphragmatic breathing.
2. Continuous breathing. The computer alerts you if you hold your breath more than 1/3 of a second.
3. Gradual exhalation, as opposed to the rapid, uncontrolled exhalation associated with stuttering.
4. Pre-voice exhalation, or letting a little air out before you begin tensing your vocal folds.
5. Gentle onset, or gradually increasing vocal volume. The computer alerts you if your vocal volume changes too rapidly. The computer also alerts you if your voice is too quiet for your air flow (which sounds breathy).
6. Continuous phonation. Breaks in vocal volume are shown on the computer monitor.
7. Adequate breath support. The computer alerts you if you continue to talk after the point at which you should take another breath.
8. Phrasing. Each of the above seven speech targets is taught first with vowels, then progressing to monosyllabic words, then to marked-length phrases.

An unpublished study of the CAFET program with 197 adults and teenagers reported that 82% met fluency criteria six months after completing the program; 89% were fluent after twelve months; and 92% were fluent two years post-therapy.

EMG and Vocal Frequency Biofeedback

In 1994 I had an idea. What if I added biofeedback to my company's DAF/FAF devices? The devices would display the user's vocal fold tension with a row of green, yellow, and red lights. When the red lights switched on, indicating the speech-production muscle tension that precedes stuttering, the device would switch on DAF/FAF to induce slower, relaxed speech. When the user's speech-production muscles relaxed, indicating fluent speech, the DAF/FAF would switch off.

I used an electromyograph (EMG) with electrodes taped to my jaw and throat. I went to a speech-language pathology convention and demonstrated the device eight hours a day for three and a half days to hundreds of speech-language pathologists. After the convention I couldn't stutter for a week. Eventually my stuttering returned, but not as severely. If I used the biofeedback device every day on telephone calls, I was fluent the rest of the day. This was my biggest breakthrough in fluency.

The secret to my success was that I was talking all day, every day, using target speech behaviors in every conversation. That a biofeedback device was helping me stay on target was important but secondary.

The DAF/FAF was tertiary. Most of the time the device had the auditory feedback switched off, indicating that my speech-production muscles were relaxed.

EMG biofeedback was effective for me but was expensive and cumbersome, with wires everywhere. I then noticed that when the green lights were on (indicating relaxed speech-production muscles) my vocal pitch was lower. I built a biofeedback device that measured my vocal frequency. This worked better than the EMG biofeedback, and was much simpler and less expensive. Since 1995 Casa Futura Technologies has made devices with DAF, FAF, and *vocal tension biofeedback.*

Efficacy Studies

A rigorous study followed 42 stutterers through the three-week program at the Institute for Stuttering Therapy and Treatment (ISTAR) in Edmonton, Alberta, Canada.[37] The fluency shaping program was based on slow, prolonged speech, starting with 1.5-seconds-per-syllable stretch, and ending with slow-normal speech. The program also works on reducing fears and avoidances, discussing stuttering openly, and changing social habits to increase speaking. The program includes a maintenance program for practicing at home. The program reduced stuttering from about 15-20% stuttered syllables to 1-2% stuttered syllables. Twelve to 24 months after therapy, about 70% of the stutterers had satisfactory fluency. About 5% were marginally successful. About 25% had unsatisfactory fluency.

The section "SLPs vs. Parents vs. Computers," (page 130) describes a large study of fluency shaping therapy with EMG biofeedback.[38]

After completion of another "smooth speech" fluency shaping stuttering therapy program, about 95% of subjects were "very satisfied" or "satisfied" with their speech at the end of the treatment. A year later, their satisfaction dropped to 43%.[39]

Another study reported that 100% of subjects who completed a year-long "prolonged speech" fluency shaping stuttering therapy program were able to speak nearly fluently. But two-thirds of the stutterers who started the program didn't complete it.[40]

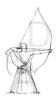

Beyond Fluency Shaping

Fluency shaping stuttering therapy was developed before much was known about motor learning and control. Some speech clinics have not refined their therapy programs to reflect advances in the field.

Improving Cognitive Stage Speech Motor Learning

In the first or *cognitive* stage of motor learning, you observe an instructor performing a motor skill that is new to you.

But speech-language pathologists may be the wrong people to model fluent speech motor skills. When learning a new motor skill, novices learn best by observing another novice making mistakes, then getting it right.

In contrast, observing a skilled person perform the task flawlessly doesn't do you much good. For example, millions of people watch Michael Jordan play basketball. Few of those people could go out on a basketball court and repeat his moves. The exceptions are people who are already skilled and want to get better, e.g., college basketball players can improve their game by watching the pros.

A stutterer watching a speech-language pathologist model gentle onsets or pull-outs is like Joe Sixpack watching Michael Jordan. The stutterer might learn more if the speech-language pathologist modeled the mistakes her other clients have made, and then showed how to correct those mistakes. Or the speech-language pathologist could prepare a video of her previous clients making mistakes, and then learning to correct their mistakes.

Improving Associative Stage Speech Motor Learning

In the second or *associative* stage of motor learning, you learn to perform and refine a new motor skill. But are there better fluent speech motor skills than the skills taught in fluency shaping stuttering therapy programs?

Lower Vocal Pitch

Speaking at a lower vocal pitch requires relaxing one's vocal folds, and reduces stuttering.[41] Unlike other fluency-enhancing techniques such as a slow speaking rate or gentle onsets, listeners like the sound of a lower vocal pitch. A lower vocal pitch communicates confidence and relaxed authority. Some listeners even say that a lower vocal pitch sounds "sexy." Speaking with a lower vocal pitch makes one feel relaxed and confident. Yet this technique is not a target behavior in fluency shaping stuttering therapy programs.

According to multichannel processing theory, performing two tasks is easier if you integrate the tasks. For example, dancing while playing the saxophone is easier than playing tennis while playing the sax. Using fluency shaping motor skills while paying attention to a conversation should be easier if the motor skills relate to the conversation. If you're trying to communicate that you're relaxed and confident, then using a "slow normal" speaking rate with a lower vocal pitch should be easier than using gentle onsets.

This technique can be trained by using relaxed, diaphragmatic breathing while feeling (with your fingers or your throat) and/or listening to your vocal fold vibrations. Begin by humming or saying "ahhhh." Bring the pitch up, then down, then up again, then down further. Repeat until your feel and hear yourself humming at a very low pitch. Now speak slowly, stretching vowels, while keeping your vocal pitch low.

Notice that your vocal volume drops as you lower your vocal pitch. Don't try to speak loudly with a low vocal pitch, you may damage your vocal folds. A lower vocal volume is usually acceptable unless you're speaking in a noisy environment or to a person with hearing loss.

Frequency-shifted auditory feedback (FAF) induces a lower vocal pitch in non-stutterers.[42] One study tested whether a half-octave FAF downshift changes stutterers' vocal pitch. The results were negative,[43] but I believe that a greater frequency shift, combined with the headphones we use today, would have positive results. In other words, if you have an FAF device, set it for one-half or one octave down, and use the best-quality headphones you have. Then say "ahhhh" or speak slowly with stretched vowels, trying to slow your vocal fold vibrations to match the frequency you hear in the headphones.

Lower vocal pitch may be difficult for women speech-language pathologists to model, or for children or women stutterers to use (Lauren Bacall might contradict that statement!). Adult men are more capable of lowering their vocal pitch. Listen to an audio book read by a male actor and then listen to another audio book read by a female actor: you'll likely hear that the male actor can perform a wider variety and range of character voices.

Automatic, Effortless Fluency

The third or *autonomous* stage of motor learning moves you from closed-loop motor control to open-loop motor control. In stuttering therapy, the autonomous stage makes fluent speech automatic and effortless.

Autonomous stage motor learning results from:

1. Practicing target muscle movements *faster* and *harder*,
2. While making *no errors,*
3. In *stressful* situations,
4. With an ideal *practice schedule,*
5. For about three million *repetitions.*

For example, you take tennis lessons. Your coach shows you

how to grip the racket properly, and swing at the ball. At first you execute this movement slowly, with little force. As your skill improves, you swing faster, and hit the ball harder. Whenever you make a mistake, your coach stops you and makes you begin again, slowly. At first your coach hits you easy balls. Then he hits harder balls to you, making the game stressful. Then you play tennis regularly. Over several years your game improves.

Where Stuttering Therapy Fails

Most stuttering therapy programs do little to train autonomous motor learning:

1.   Your speech-language pathologist tells you to make a conscious effort to speak fluently. You're told that if your fluency fails, it's your fault for not concentrating on your speech.
2.   All practice is done with relaxed speech-production muscles. You never increase muscle tension.
3.   All practice is done at slow speaking rates.
4.   All practice is done in the speech clinic, or at home alone. You don't do practice in high-stress situations.

Increasing Force and Speed

Stuttering therapy programs fail to train the autonomous stage of speech motor learning because of a counterintuitive aspect of stuttering. Stuttering is characterized by excessive speech-production muscle activity. The obvious but wrong treatment for stuttering is to reduce speech-production muscle activity, i.e., to speak with relaxed breathing, vocal folds, and articulation muscles.

As noted earlier (page 38), speech-language pathologists see that slowing down and using closed-loop speech motor control eliminates stuttering. They reach the obvious but wrong conclusion that stuttering therapy should be done at slow speaking rates.

Fluency shaping therapy begins by training slow, relaxed, fluent speech motor skills. Similarly, golf and tennis instruction begins with slow, relaxed, correct movements. Golf and tennis instructors then have you increase your force and speed. In contrast, speech-language pathologists tell you not to increase your force and speed. It may seem counterintuitive, but after you master slow, relaxed fluent speech, you must increase both the speed and force of your speech, without making errors, to train automatic, effortless fluency.

Increasing Force

The force of your speech is measured by volume. Work on getting loud. But don't shout or yell. Instead, *project* your voice. Vocal volume is a factor of both exhalation volume and vocal fold tension. Increase your exhalation volume while keeping your vocal folds relatively relaxed. This result is high volume with the intonations of normal conversational speech. Stage actors do this.

Increase your onset speed while maintaining long syllable duration. Pretend that your forearm is a sports car's accelerator. When your fist is up, your vocal volume is quiet. As you push your fist down, your volume increases. When your fist is all the way down, you're at maximum volume. Listeners one hundred feet away should hear you.

Slowly lower your fist to produce a gentle onset. Then slam your fist down fast to go from silence to maximum volume. Then hold that volume while stretching the vowel. Pull your fist up fast to end the word with speed. This is slow speech with maximum effort.

Be careful not to damage your vocal folds. Stop if you feel hoarse or start to lose your voice.

Increasing Speed

Shorten syllable duration from two seconds, to one second, to one-half second, to one-quarter second. Practice this both with relaxed, quiet speech, and with loud, forceful speech.

Using the practice word lists (page 175) say each word four times:

1. Slow and relaxed (quietly).
2. Slow and projecting your voice (loudly).
3. Relaxed (quietly) with a quick onset.
4. Loudly projecting the word with a hard onset.

Where to Practice Force and Speed

It's hard to practice loud speech in a small room. The ideal place to practice is an empty auditorium. Have your speech-language pathologist sit in the back row. Stand on stage and project your voice to her. She yells, "Can't hear you!" until you reach ideal volume.

Another place to practice is near a building that produces an echo. A third place to practice is on a freeway overpass. Demosthenes, the stutterer who became the greatest orator of ancient Greece, projected his voice over breaking waves at the seashore. Work on projecting your voice over the waves of traffic.

Reinforcing On-Target Speech

Increasing speed and force *myelinates* or reinforces neural pathways in your brain. A mistake reinforces the wrong neural pathways.

Learning to talk fluently requires talking fluently 100% of the time. That sounds like circular advice, and it is. Reinforcing motor skills is a "virtuous cycle." Using target skills reinforces the skills, making the skills easier to use.

Conversely, stuttering reinforces undesirable speech motor skills (core behaviors, page 8) and bad communication habits (secondary behaviors, page 8). Stuttering sets up a "vicious cycle" instead of a "virtuous cycle."

Swimming Analogy

I wanted to improve my swimming. At first I could swim only one length of the pool, and then I had to rest. But I got in the pool three times a week. I found that a small flotation device helped me swim five or ten laps. After two months something "clicked" in my brain and I swam half a mile. It was easy, almost effortless. I didn't need the flotation device any more.

Then I moved to a building without a swimming pool, stopped swimming, and now I swim as poorly as I did before that summer.

Similarly, stutterers go to speech therapy three times a week for months. Then suddenly one day they find themselves talking fluently, without effort. If they discontinue speech therapy, this "lucky" fluency disappears and they go back to stuttering.

Stutterers' brains have two sets of speech motor programs (see the chapter "Responding to Stress," page 76). Sometimes our brains pick the fluent speech motor programs. At other times our brains pick the stuttering speech motor programs. Speech therapy reinforces the fluent speech motor programs. Eventually this fluent speech becomes habitual. But during "lucky" fluency this habit is precariously balanced. One stressful day, in which you allow yourself to stutter, can reinforce the stuttering motor programs, and your "lucky" fluency is gone.

Speech Buddies

Children learn grammar by listening to other people talking, then speaking, then having their parents correct their grammar. You may not remember this, but after a vacation to the seashore you said, "We went nearly to the beach every day," and your mother corrected you, "No, dear, we went to the beach nearly every day."

Your mom was your speech buddy. You need another speech buddy now, to help you correct your speech when you're dysfluent.

Ask your speech-language pathologist to let you organize a practice group with her other clients. Meet once a week to practice fluent speech. Exchange telephone numbers and arrange to call a speech buddy every day.

Here's an idea that'll get you talking fluently. If you have a spare bedroom in your house, call your local university and offer to let a speech-language pathology student live rent-free, in return for reminding you to use fluency shaping skills. If you don't live near a university, call your school district and see if they have a speech-language pathologist who'd go for free rent.

Train your spouse, housemates, and the people you work with to remind you to use fluency skills. If you're a parent with a child in speech therapy, ask your child's speech-language pathologist to train you to correct your child at home (see "SLPs vs. Parents vs. Computers," (page 130).

Bring your spouse or housemates to speech therapy. Ask them to give you a warning sign when you don't use your fluency targets, and offer to pay them $1 whenever you stutter.

My Romantic Disaster of 1996

In eighth grade I had a teacher with a forceful personality and a large ego. He decided to cure my stuttering. Whenever I stuttered he stopped me, then told me to say it without stuttering. I hadn't had speech therapy and had no idea what to do. His method was as effective as teaching me Chinese by stopping me from speaking English and telling me to speak in Chinese.

Twenty years later I'd completed several speech therapy programs. I'd used electronic anti-stuttering devices for several years. I dated a woman who disliked my stuttering. Whenever I started to block, she'd give me a certain look. I'd stop, relax my breathing and vocal folds, and speak fluently.

Within a few days with her I was talking fluently all the time. The relationship crashed and burned shortly after that.

For an individual who hasn't completed a speech therapy program, a person pointing out their stuttering is the worst thing. Such an individual doesn't have any control over his speech. Telling him to talk fluently increases his stress and his stuttering.

But for an individual who has mastered fluent speech skills, pointing out his disfluencies and reminding him to use fluent speech skills will help him. When you're at that stage, find someone to do this for you. (See the section "Modeling," page 126.)

Start a Virtuous Cycle

Do whatever you need to get into the virtuous cycle. You may have to do things that are difficult or embarrassing—e.g., telling your co-workers that you stutter (hint: they've probably already figured that out!).

Once you're in a virtuous cycle, fluent speech will become easier and easier with less and less effort. The difficult things will become easier, and the embarrassing things won't be embarrassing (or necessary). If you've done it right, you'll only have to do these things for a few days or weeks.

Getting into a virtuous cycle may require:

1. Using closed-loop speech motor control (slow speech).
2. Using an electronic anti-stuttering device.
3. Taking a dopamine-antagonist medication.
4. Talking in uncomfortable situations, e.g., to strangers or to telemarketers.

For a high-testosterone kickstart, see "The *Predator* Approach" (page 87).

Practicing Under Stress

Autonomous motor learning requires practicing a new motor skill in stressful situations.

Design a hierarchy of stressful situations. The first might be leaving a message on your speech-language pathologist's answering machine. When you can do that comfortably and fluently, you might talk to telemarketers using closed-loop speech motor control (slow, fluent speech). Then you could join Toastmasters and make a series of speeches to your club. More about this in the chapter "Responding to Stress" (page 76).

Practice Scheduling

The United States Postal Service studied workers learning to operate mail-sorting machines (similar to typewriters). All subjects received 60 hours of training. The scheduling varied among four groups.

One group had two two-hour sessions per day, for 15 days. A second group had one two-hour session per day, for 30 days. A third group had two one-hour sessions per day, for 30 days. The fourth group had one one-hour session per day, for 60 days.

The first group (two two-hour sessions per day) learned fastest, but in the long run had the worst performance. The fourth group (one one-hour session per day) took the longest to get "up to speed," but eventually had the best performance.

Surprisingly, the postal workers preferred the two-hour/two-session schedule, even though they had the worst performance. People are impatient. They don't want to spend 60 days learning something, if they think there's a 15-day shortcut.

Extinguishing Old Skills

We could simplistically conclude that you should practice stuttering therapy no more than one hour per day. But there's an essential difference between speech therapy and mail sorting. The postal workers were learning a new motor skill. Stutterers have to learn a new motor skill and extinguish an old motor skill. As noted earlier, coaches often prefer to work with individuals who have never played a sport and haven't learned bad habits, rather than work with experienced athletes and have to break their bad habits.

To extinguish an old motor skill you must stop doing it. Perhaps the ideal stuttering therapy is done one hour per day, and then you take a vow of silence the rest of the day. But that's unrealistic. To burn new fluent neural pathways, and extinguish old stuttering neural pathways, you must use fluent speech every time you talk. You must never stutter. Each disfluency weakens your new fluent neural pathways and strengthens your old stuttering neural pathways.

Extinguishing a maladaptive motor skill isn't the same as "breaking" a bad habit. Maladaptive motor skills enable you to perform a desirable behavior, but not as a well as a better motor skill. For example, touchtyping is better than two-fingered typing, but two-fingered typing also gets the job done. In contrast, picking my nose is an undesirable behavior. I wish that a teacher had taught me to touchtype when I was a child. I don't wish that a teacher had taught me a better way to pick my nose.

Because maladaptive motor skills enable you to perform a desirable behavior, it's hard to unlearn them and replace them with optimal motor skills. Stuttering isn't like picking your nose. Your mother could slap your hand and stop you whenever you pick your nose. If she stopped you every time you stuttered, you wouldn't be able to talk.

Extinguishing a maladaptive motor skill may involve "one step forward, one step back" temporarily. To speak fluently, you may have to speak much slower, or not respond immediately while you focus on your speech motor skills.

Intensive Residential Speech Therapy Programs

Some stutterers go to intensive residential speech therapy programs. These programs typically last three weeks. You're surrounded by speech-language pathologists and other stutterers, and isolated from the real world. For the first two weeks, you use two-second stretch all the time. In the third week, you move to one-second stretch, then half-second, and finally quarter-second slow normal.

Intensive residential speech therapy programs are like the postal workers who did the "short cut" training. In three weeks of intensive therapy you learn to talk fluently. But many stutterers find that long-term results are disappointing.

Your Ideal Practice Schedule

Work with your speech-language pathologist to develop a practice schedule. A severe stutterer may have to spend many hours a day doing "homework."

Don't practice sitting alone in a room reading endless word lists. This isn't going to produce carryover fluency to stressful situations.

A one-hour daily practice could have the following elements:

- After breakfast, twenty minutes of high intensity practice (projection and hard onsets), with practice word lists (page 175).
- During the day, a stressful twenty-minute session while using a biofeedback device to keep your vocal folds relaxed. This could be calling strangers for your job.
- After supper, twenty minutes of very slow closed-loop speech motor control conversation. Call another stutterer in your support group. Or call infomercial toll-free numbers.

How Long Does Autonomous Learning Take?

Gymnasts practice daily for about eight years to become proficient.

Motor learning researchers studied the manual (hand) skills of cigar-makers.[44] Beginner cigar-makers worked three times slower than experienced cigar-makers. Becoming fully skilled required making three million cigars.

Three million repetitions were also needed for Japanese pearl handlers to become proficient. The Suzuki method of teaching violin to children requires the production of about 2.5 million notes. Basketball, football, and baseball throws require about a million practice throws.

This suggests that making fluent speech automatic and effortless requires saying about three million syllables. At five syllables per second, talking four hours a day (just your time talking, not combined talking and listening), you could produce three million syllables in six weeks.

If you got a job answering telephone calls, and you did your stuttering therapy skills on every call, and you connected a biofeedback device into your telephone to alert you when you missed a therapy target, and you spent your free time at Toastmasters clubs making speeches or volunteering at a hospital's information desk, fluent speech might become automatic for you in six weeks.

But most stutterers practice between ten minutes and one hour per day. If they were silent the rest of the day, they'd say three million syllables somewhere between six months and three years.

No one has studied whether using undesirable motor skills cancels out on-target practice. In other words, does a half-hour of on-target practice get cancelled out by not using fluency skills the rest of the day? Such a practice schedule might take years to produce automatic fluent speech—or might never work.

Zen in the Art of Stuttering

> Zen is the "everyday mind," as was proclaimed by Baso (died 788); this "everyday mind" is no more than "sleeping when tired, eating when hungry." As soon as we reflect, deliberate, and conceptualize, the original unconsciousness is lost and a thought interferes. We no longer eat while eating, we no longer sleep while sleeping. The arrow is off the string but does not fly straight to the target...Calculation which is miscalculation sets in...The archer's confused mind betrays itself in every direction and every field of activity.
> — Daisetz T. Suzuki, intro to *Zen in the Art of Archery*

> Stuttering is what you do trying not to stutter again.
> — Wendell Johnson

The goal of stuttering therapy is spontaneous fluent speech. The goal of Zen is to do life activities without self-conscious calculating and thinking.

Non-stutterers usually talk without self-conscious calculating and thinking. But sometimes they are self-conscious about their speech. Fear of public speaking is common. And non-stutterers are self-conscious about asking the boss for a raise, or asking someone out on a date, or when discussing an embarrassing subject. Speech pathologists call this *pragmatics*—the mental effort of calculating the listener's reaction to your speech. In the Zen framework, pragmatics is the calculation that is miscalculation.

A goal of stuttering therapy could be to become a "Zen master of speech," just as other Zen masters are archers or swordsmen or calligraphers. To make an analogy to Baso, you sleep when tired, eat when hungry, and talk when you need to communicate. You don't worry about the listener's reaction. You don't fear embarrassment. If the listener doesn't do what you want or expect, you don't get upset.

You also talk fluently—but let's define fluency as if we're learning a foreign language. You need vocabulary to express your thoughts, grammar so your meaning isn't misconstrued, and accent and articulation to be understood. Mild stuttering may be OK, if your listener understands you, and you don't fear or avoid speaking. Van Riper called this "fluent stuttering," and a Zen master might call it "fluency which is not fluency."

Eugen Herrigel and Awa Kenzo

Eugen Herrigel (1884–1955) was a German professor of philosophy, with a special interest in mysticism. From 1924 to 1929 he taught philosophy in Japan, and studied archery with an eccentric archery instructor named Awa Kenzo. Awa taught archery as a mystical religion, called *Daishadokyo*. Daishadokyo had nothing to do with Zen Buddhism or the traditional Japanese art of archery (*kyudo* or *kyujutsu*).[45] In 1936, Herrigel wrote a 20-page essay about his experiences, and then in 1948 expanded the essay into a short book entitled *Zen in the Art of Archery*. Regardless of whether it accurately portrays Zen Buddhism or traditional Japanese archery, the book has many accurate insights into motor learning and control. For example, a central theme of the book is that a complex and difficult motor skill seems to be mentally and physically effortless after years of practice, and that the motor skill is best performed when your body seems to execute the motor skill without your mind's conscious control. The book is wonderfully written and has been a bestseller for more than fifty years, in many languages.

Master Awa's first lesson was drawing the bow, letting "only your two hands do the work, while your arm and shoulder muscles remain relaxed, as though they looked on impassively."

This step is like stuttering therapy, with the goal of speaking while keeping your speech-production muscles relaxed.

Herrigel couldn't do this first step. He would "start trembling after a few moments, and my breathing became more and more labored." Sounds like stuttering!

He was trying to draw a six-foot bow held above his head, which requires great strength. But somehow the Master did this effortlessly.

> ...he called out to me to "Relax! Relax!"...the day came when...I lost patience and brought myself to admit that I absolutely could not draw the bow in the manner pre-scribed.
>
> "You cannot do it," explained the Master, "because you do not breathe right."

Sounds like stuttering therapy! The Master continued,

> "Press your breath down gently after breathing in, so that the abdominal wall is tightly stretched, and hold it there for a while. Then breathe out as slowly and evenly as possible, and after a short pause, draw a quick breath of air again—out and in continually, in a rhythm, that will gradually settle itself. If it is done properly, you will feel the shooting becoming easier every day. For through this breathing you will not only discover the source of all spiritual strength but will also cause this source to flow more abundantly, and to pour more easily through your limbs the more relaxed you are."
>
> And as if to prove it, he drew his strong bow and in-vited me to step behind him and feel his arm muscles. They were indeed quite relaxed, as though they were doing no work at all.
>
> The new way of breathing was practiced, without bow and arrow at first, until it came naturally. The slight feel-

ing of discomfort noticeable in the beginning was quickly overcome. The Master attached so much importance to breathing out as slowly and steadily as possible to the very end, that, for better practice and control, he made us combine it with a humming note.

First relaxed breathing, and now vocal fold vibration!

I cannot think back to those days without recalling, over and over again, how difficult I found it, in the beginning, to get my breathing to work out right...

When, to excuse myself, I once remarked that I was conscientiously making an effort to keep relaxed, he replied: "That's just the trouble, you make an effort to think about it. Concentrate entirely on your breathing, as if you had nothing else to do!"

I've heard speech-language pathologists say the same thing...

It took me considerable time before I succeeded in doing what the Master wanted. But—I succeeded. I learned to lose myself so effortlessly in the breathing that I sometimes had the feeling that I myself was not breathing but—strange as this may sound—being breathed. And even when, in hours of thoughtful reflection, I struggled against this bold idea, I could no longer doubt that the breathing held out all that the Master had promised.

Learning to draw the bow took a year. Perhaps stuttering therapies are unsuccessful because we expect results too quickly. Imagine stuttering therapy starting with a year of breathing exercises!

Then Herrigel learned to loose the arrow. This was even more difficult than drawing the bow. Herrigel kept jerking his hand at the moment of release, which resulted in "visible shaking of my whole body and affected the bow and arrow as well." This caused the arrow to "wobble."

The Master told Herrigel, "Don't think of what you have to do, don't consider how to carry it out! You mustn't open the right hand on purpose."

Herrigel told the Master that after drawing the bow, "unless the shot comes at once I shan't be able to endure the tension…I can't wait any longer."

The Master replied that Herrigel's inability to wait was because, "You do not wait for fulfillment, but brace yourself for failure."

Herrigel spent three years learning to release the arrow. The Master kept saying to release the arrow without tension, like a bamboo leaf holding snow, bending lower and lower until the snow slips off. The bamboo leaf waits without effort until the snow falls off.

In stuttering therapy, the first word of a phrase should be without effort, rolling off your vocal folds like the snow sliding off the bamboo leaf. You shouldn't intend to say the first word, as the archer doesn't open his hand on purpose. The word should say itself, without your planning or calculating or trying.

Herrigel's three years practice releasing the arrow suggests that learning to release the first word of a phrase may also take three years, and be the hardest part of stuttering therapy.

Herrigel was dedicated to his practice, but he couldn't release the arrow smoothly. The Master kept telling Herrigel to become "truly egoless." Herrigel became dejected, and planned to discontinue the archery lessons, concluding that, "all my efforts of the last few years had become meaningless."

Then, one day, after a shot, the Master made a deep bow and broke off the lesson. "Just then 'It' shot!" he cried.

"It" meant that Herrigel had loosed a shot without loosing the shot. "It" had loosed the shot, not Herrigel. The Master could not say anymore what "It" was, just that "It" can only be known through experience.

Only after considerable time did more right shots occasionally come off, which the Master signaled by a deep

bow. How it happened that they loosed themselves without my doing anything, how it came about that my tightly
closed right hand suddenly flew back wide open, I could
not explain then and I cannot explain today...I got to the
point of being able to distinguish, on my own, the right
shots from the failures. The qualitative difference is so
great that it cannot be overlooked once it has been experienced.

In stuttering therapy, the difference between your relaxed, fluent
voice and your tense, stuttering voice is as obvious as night and
day—after you learn relaxed, fluent speech. Until then it seems
impossible.

The Master then began training Herrigel to shoot at a target,
adding, "He who has a hundred miles to walk should reckon ninety
as half the journey."

The Master refused to teach Herrigel to aim, insisting that the
target was not the goal, and the goal cannot be aimed at, and that
the goal doesn't have a name, except maybe "enlightenment."

But even though the Master did not aim, all of his shots lodged
in the black center of the target, from sixty feet away.

At first Herrigel tried to shoot without caring if the arrows hit
the target. But he couldn't do this, and "I confessed to him that I
was at the end of my tether."

The Master replied:

You worry yourself unnecessarily. Put the thought of hitting right out of your mind! You can be a Master even if
every shot does not hit.

Remember that you can be a Zen master of speech even if you
still stutter.

When the Master said he sees "the goal as though I don't see
it," Herrigel replied that the Master should then be able to shoot
blindfolded. The Master then had Herrigel set up the target in
darkness, except for one candle. Herrigel could not see the target at
all, but the Master shot two arrows. When Herrigel turned on the

lights, he saw that not only had both arrows hit the bulls-eye, but the second arrow had hit the first and splintered it!

Herrigel describes the following months as the hardest yet, of trying to hit the target yet not trying to hit the target. He gradually came to see the value of this training:

> It destroyed the last traces of any preoccupation with myself and the fluctuations of my mood.

Finally, the Master had Herrigel shoot in front of spectators, and awarded him a diploma, "inscribed with the degree of mastery." Before Herrigel returned to Europe, the Master added,

> I must only warn you of one thing. You have become a different person in the course of these years. For this is what the art of archery means: a profound and far-reaching contest of the archer with himself. Perhaps you have hardly noticed it yet, but you will feel it very strongly when you meet your friends and acquaintances again...You will see with other eyes and measure with other measures.

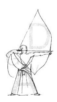

Responding to Stress

Under stress, people's voices change. They tense their speech-production muscles, increasing vocal pitch. They talk faster. They repeat words or phrases. They add interjections, such as "uh." These are *normal dysfluencies*. A study[46] found that under stress, non-stutterers went from 0% to 4% dysfluencies. Stutterers went from 1% to 9%.

The "conventional wisdom" is that stutterers are always nervous or stressed out. Many psychological studies have proven that this isn't true. But stress has an important role in stuttering.

All stutterers can talk fluently. In relaxed, low-stress situations we can say any sound or word fluently. If you're a severe stutterer, there might not be many such situations. But there are some.

In other situations we stutter. How many paraplegics do you know who can walk in some situations, but not other situations? Or blind persons who can't see certain people, but clearly see others? OK, that describes young women after I turned 40, but most blind people are blind all the time.

Our brains are capable of producing fluent speech. We have all the speech motor programs necessary to produce any speech sound, fluently.

We also have speech motor programs for producing dysfluent sounds. Stutterers have two sets of open-loop speech motor programs (see page 31). Our brains *select* one or the other set of speech motor programs, depending on *environmental cues*—where we are or whom we're talking to.

This is like a person who grew up summers in Vermont and winters in Georgia. Such a person would have a set of speech motor programs to speak with a New England accent. And this person would have a set of speech motor programs to speak with a

Southern accent. When she's in Vermont, hearing people speak with New England accents, her brain automatically selects the New England accent speech motor programs. In Georgia, her brain selects Southern accent speech motor programs.

You always have choices for handling stressful situations. Some choices trigger your brain to automatically select dysfluent speech motor programs. Other choices trigger your brain to select fluent speech motor programs. This chapter will teach you to make choices for handling stress that automatically select fluent, relaxed speech. You'll feel relaxed and speak confidently even when non-stutterers are stressed out.

Are Responses to Stress Psychological?

According to "conventional wisdom," stuttering is a psychological disorder because stutterers speak fluently in low-stress situations and stutter in high-stress situations.

But many responses to stress are physical. For example, "fight or flight" increases heart rate. Stress is considered to be a factor in the development of physical disorders, such as heart disease and gastrointestinal disorders. Why is stuttering considered to be a psychological disorder, but heart disease is considered to be a physical disorder?

This chapter presents stuttering a response to stress, and then presents strategies for better handling stress. Although the presented strategies might be termed "psychological," I object to referring to responses to stress as psychological responses. You can treat responses to stress physically, such as with medications or using an anti-stuttering device. I've put those treatments into other chapters. Perhaps more than the other factors, responses to stress show that the factors that contribute to stuttering are complex and interconnected.

Stuttering Reduces Stress

Systolic blood pressure is an indicator of stress. Stuttering reduced stutterers' blood pressure 10%.[47] In contrast, fluent speech, chewing gum, and sitting quietly each reduced blood pressure about 2%.

You're thinking, "No way. Stuttering doesn't relax me. Stuttering doesn't feel like a massage and warm bath."

But think about it. Stutterers are, on average, disfluent on 10% of syllables. We say 90% of syllables fluently. But we don't say one hundred syllables fluently, and then finish a conversation with ten dysfluencies. Stuttering usually occurs on the first sound of the first word, in a stressful situation. In other words, your stress builds up as you anticipate speaking. You stutter, and this releases stress. You then say several syllables fluently.

You then stutter on another syllable, then say several more syllables fluently. Usually your speech improves over the course of the conversation, and your last few sentences are your most fluent.

If your blood pressure were monitored in such a conversation, it might look like this (this is speculative, not based on research):

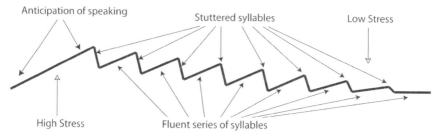

Figure 11: Stuttering Reducing Stress

Your stress increases as you anticipate speaking. You block on the first syllable. This reduces your stress, and you speak fluently. Your stress builds up again, and you stutter again. This reduces your stress, and the cycle repeats until you're speaking fluently at the end of the conversation.

Stuttering Isn't a Good Response to Stress

Stuttering doesn't change the stressful situation. For example, a highway patrol officer pulls you over for speeding. Stuttering won't make the officer think you weren't speeding.

Stuttering might make the situation worse. For example, the

highway patrol officer mistakes your stuttering for methampheta-mine addiction. He handcuffs you and searches your car. This stresses you more, and you stutter more.

Stuttering and stress are a vicious cycle. Stuttering reduces your stress for a few seconds, but then causes more stress. You get stuck in the cycle, unable to break free.

Another study measured *listeners'* systolic blood pressure.[48] Listening to stuttering made listeners feel stress. The listeners' increased stress may in turn increase the stutterer's stress. Again, stuttering and stress start a vicious cycle.

This chapter will show you that you have other choices for han-dling stress, instead of stuttering. These other choices reduce stress, instead of throwing you into an endless cycle.

Distraction and Placebos

A Ph.D. speech-language pathologist wrote, "Distraction methods can be used to eliminate stuttering temporarily."[49] The scientific term for "distraction" is *dual-tasking*. For example, psychologists test cognitive impairment by having a subject count strings of tones while looking for symbols in a Yellow Pages directory.

If distractions eliminated stuttering, then stutterers would dual-task when they wanted to talk fluently, perhaps by working a Rubik's cube or playing a pocket video game. Two studies investi-gated this. In the first study, stutterers stepped on and off a 10-inch platform while reading out loud. In the second study, stutterers manually tracked an irregular line on a rotating drum while speak-ing. Neither distraction was able to reduce stuttering.[50]

Dual-tasking can make stuttering worse. Every stutterer who has completed a fluency shaping therapy course knows that you can focus on *what* you're saying or on *how* you're talking, but doing both at the same time is a challenge. In other words, using fluency shaping skills in a clinical environment is easy, but the distractions of conversations make using fluency shaping skills difficult.

Beliefs and Placebos

A Ph.D. speech-language pathologist wrote, "if a stutterer were to forget that he was a stutterer, he would have no further difficulty with his speech."[51] Another Ph.D. speech-language pathologist wrote, "our beliefs about stuttering seem to be one of the main factors in stuttering severity."[52]

These hypotheses have been repeatedly proven wrong—but not in studies set up for that purpose. Instead, studies of medications to treat stuttering are usually *placebo-controlled*. A placebo is a pill without a medication. The purpose of a placebo is to make study subjects believe that they are getting medication that will treat their disease or disorder. In other words, study subjects are all told that they will receive a medication that might (or might not) reduce their stuttering, but only half the subjects get the medication. The other half get the placebo pills. The latter are perfect subjects for testing the hypothesis that believing you won't stutter will lead you to not stutter.

A study found that placebos did not reduce stuttering.[53] Another study also found that placebos had no effect on stuttering—but the placebos caused terrible side effects![54] Reported placebo side effects included constipation, sexual dysfunction, dizziness, sweating, and tremors. The placebo produced six times more side effects than the medication in the study.

This raises an interesting question. Placebos are effective treatments for almost every disease and symptom:

> Study after study showed that, for virtually any disease, a substantial portion of symptoms—roughly one-third, by most estimates—would improve when patients were given a placebo treatment with no pharmacological activity. Patients simply believed that the treatment would help them, and somehow, it did.[55]

> ...for a wide range of afflictions, including pain, high blood pressure, asthma and cough, roughly 30 to 40 percent of patients experience relief after taking a placebo...placebos seem to be most reliably effective for

afflictions in which stress directly affects the symptoms...pain, asthma and moderate high blood pressure
can become worse when the patient is upset...placebos
may work in part by lessening the apprehension associated with the disease [because] the immune system
falters under stressful conditions.[56]

Stuttering may be the only disorder that placebos have no effect
upon! In other words, stuttering isn't affected by belief, and
stutterers can't be "psyched" into fluency. In contrast, heart
disease, asthma, etc. appear to be physical diseases but are actually
in large part psychological (or psychophysiological or psychoso-
matic). Could stuttering—long believed to be entirely psychological—actually have no psychological component?

Good Stress, Bad Stress

We experience many forms of stress. Some forms of stress reduce
stuttering. Other forms of stress increase stuttering. Still other
forms of stress have no effect on stuttering.

Adrenaline and Fluency-Enhancing Stress
In World War Two, a severe stutterer regularly spoke fluently for
mortar communication during combat.[57]

One night, a person physically threatened me for several hours.
I've never been so fluent in my life! My voice was calm and
relaxed as I tried to get the person to calm down.

Noradrenaline and adrenaline compete with dopamine for the
binding sites on D4 receptors, and when bound, act as agonists. At
the same time, through feedback inhibition, norepinephrine inhibits
tyrosine hydroxylase, which in turn inhibits the production of
dopamine. Because dopamine in the striatal system increases
stuttering (see "Anti-Stuttering Medications," page 100), and
adrenaline blocks dopamine, "fight or flight" situations that increase adrenaline reduce stuttering.[58]

Stutterers report that when the adrenaline wears off, their stuttering increases.[59]

Physiological Stress

Physical activities such as running or bicycling elevate heart rate, blood pressure, etc. Dropping a rock on your foot is another form of physiological stress.

Exercise makes you breathe harder, with your diaphragm. If your stuttering involves disordered breathing you may stutter more when exercising. On the other hand, if your speech-language pathologist trained you to speak with diaphragmatic breathing, exercise may improve your fluency.

In general, physiological stress has no effect on stuttering.

Progressive relaxation trains you to relax all of your muscles, starting with your toes and ending with your facial muscles. Progressive relaxation has minimal effect on stuttering. Relaxation exercises only reduce stuttering when the focus is on relaxing speech production muscles (respiration, vocal folds, and the lips, jaw, and tongue articulators).

Cognitive Stress

Hearing or seeing several things at once, especially if the events contradict each other (*cognitive dissonance*), increases stuttering.

For example, I can't stand talking to a person who's watching television. Or a person who's playing guitar, or picks up the phone to make a call while I'm trying to talk to him. I have a cousin who watches TV, plays guitar, and makes telephone calls, all at the same time, when I try to talk to him.

Listeners should give their full attention to stutterers. Turning away to do something else, even if you say, "I'm still listening," will increase the individual's stuttering.

If a listener won't give you his or her full attention, consider whether the conversation matters to you. If not, walk away.

Time Pressure

Time pressure increases stuttering. At the beginning of this chapter

I mentioned a study in which stress increased dysfluency. [60] The study began with subjects seeing "red" written in red on a computer monitor. They had to say "red." The screens came faster and faster, to increase time pressure.

Next, cognitive stress was added. For example, the word "red" was written in yellow on a computer monitor. The subjects had to say "yellow," not "red."

These results were dramatic. Non-stutterers went from 0% dysfluent words, to 2% disfluencies with time pressure, then to 4% with time pressure and cognitive stress.

Stutterers went from 1% stuttered words, to 3% with time pressure, to 9% with time pressure and cognitive stress.

Telling a stutterer to talk faster will have the opposite effect. Instead, tell stutterers to take all the time they need.

Use time pressure to your advantage by limiting what you say. Tell most people to make a five-minute speech and they ramble on for ten minutes, without getting to the point. If you're asked to make a five-minute speech, get to the point in one minute, without the rambling. What you think is one minute will actually take two or three minutes, and then adding in stuttering will make it five minutes. Even when I stuttered severely I had professors compliment my presentations.

Pragmatic Speech
Pragmatic speech is intended to cause another person to do a specific action. This might be telling a co-worker how to send a fax. Don't say, "Let me do it for you."

More stressful is asking someone to do something you want, when you're afraid that the person will say no. For example, asking your boss for a raise, or asking an attractive person out on a date. The listener is relatively powerful, and you're in a position of relative weakness.

To reduce stress, we usually try to make the question look casual. You "just happen" to run into the attractive person at the health club, and you "just happen" to have tickets to a show in your pocket, and you "casually" ask for a date. Or you wait until you've just landed a big sale for the company, and "jokingly" tell your boss that you deserve a raise.

But then you stutter, belying that this "casual" conversation is stressful for you. Your listener recognizes your weak position and, if he or she has an ego problem, enjoys manipulating you. A powerful person with an ego problem manipulating you is a pretty good description of stress.

Instead, use other ways to reduce stress. First, don't make a big effort to set up a "casual"-seeming situation. The more effort you make, the more stress you'll feel that it's "now or never" to get a positive response.

Next, use Winston Churchill's strategy (page 147) of preparing your points in advance ("I deserve a raise for three reasons..."), anticipating your listener's objections, and preparing responses to those objections.

Then use slow speech to explain each point. Pause between points. Use the pause to check that your breathing and vocal folds are relaxed. You'll sound confident and in control.

Lastly, be willing to walk away. Is it the end of the world if your housemate doesn't wash the dishes, or you don't get a date? Visual what you'll do and how you'll feel if the answer is no.

Be an Anti-Mirror

People tend to mirror each others' speech patterns. A person speaks fast to you, so you talk fast. A listener jumps in before you finish your sentences, so you interrupt her sentences. A person gets angry at you, so you raise your voice and get emotional.

All of those speech patterns increase stuttering. Instead, be an anti-mirror. The faster others speak, the slower you respond. Instead of interrupting, wait for the other person to finish speaking, then count to three before you start to talk. If a person expresses anger, make your voice quieter, slower, and less emotional.

Embarrassment and Uncertainty

We fear embarrassment. For example, I'm about to call you Josh, when I think, "Wait, his name is Joel."

This fear is multiplied when we're speaking to more than one person—saying something embarrassing in front of an audience of a thousand people is more embarrassing than in front of one person.

Lack of feedback increases our fears of embarrassment. In other words, when speaking on television we can't observe the reactions of listeners. You could say something stupid and never know it. You try to remember and analyze the last thing you said while you're saying something else.

If you say something embarrassing, make a joke out of it. For example, I was waiting for a woman I'd never met. She said she'd arrive at 6pm. At 6:05pm a woman parked in front of my house. I went out and said, "You must be Ariana." She didn't say anything so I said it again. She responded that she wasn't Ariana. I said, "Oh my God, I'm so embarrassed," in a humorous way.

Then there's always the "at my advanced age I can't remember names." That's funny whether you're 90 or 19.

Acknowledging embarrassment ends embarrassment.

Establishing Status

We communicate status largely via speech. We feel anxiety when status is ambiguous.

For example, you find a large, muscular hoodlum sitting on your car. Do you speak with firm authority, ordering the hoodlum off your car? Do choose a friendly, buddy-buddy tone of equality? Do you meekly ask if the hoodlum could let you have your car back?

Stuttering doesn't necessarily communicate low status. Embarrassment and anxiety about stuttering communicates low status. Calmly stuttering, while looking the hoodlum in the eye, establishes that you're not afraid to stutter and you're not afraid of the hoodlum.

Moral Stress

Whether you tell the truth or lie, you can use stuttering to make listeners believe that you're telling the truth. Interrogations start with "baseline" questions such as your name. Get into some good dysfluencies on your name.

Imagine yourself hooked up to a lie detector machine. Start the conversation with a topic unrelated to the big issue. Interrogators call these the "baseline" questions, such as asking your name. Get into some good dysfluencies. Imagine making the lie detector needle swing into the red.

Then when you're asked the big question, pause, relax your breathing and your vocal folds, and slowly and fluently tell your story—truthfully or otherwise. A lie detector machine will indicate that you're telling the truth. A human listener will do the same.

Categorize Stress to React Rationally

Movies show characters in stressful situations. When watching movies, name the type of stress a character experiences. Soon you should feel an inner voice say "moral stress," or "time pressure" when watching movies.

Then the same light bulb will switch on in your mind when watching people in daily life. When the light bulb switches on in your stressful situations, you're on your way to eliminating this type of stress.

Stress causes you to react emotionally, not rationally. When reacting emotionally, you react one way. Different people have different emotional reactions, depending on their personality type. For example, one person might react with outward anger, when another person reacts with inward shame. That doesn't matter. What matters is the automatic, single response to all stressful situations.

Shifting out of an emotion and into "neutral" enables you to see other possible responses, and select the best response. The light bulb switching on enables you to switch gears.

Speech-Related Fears and Anxieties

Introducing yourself to an attractive person. Raising your hand to answer a teacher's question. Ordering in a restaurant. Calling a store to ask if they have what you want. Making a toast at your best friend's wedding reception. Calling to order a pizza. Leaving a voicemail.

Do any of these make you nervous? Any that you never, ever do? Everyone is nervous about some speaking situations. Public speaking is humanity's most common fear, greater than the fear of death. Few women will introduce themselves to a man to ask for a date, or call a man who's given his telephone number and asked for a date. Ordering in a French restaurant is scarier than ordering at McDonald's.

The *Predator* Approach

Rent the video *Predator*, starring Arnold Schwarzenegger and Jesse Ventura. Settle down with a bowl of popcorn to watch the governor of California and the governor of Minnesota discuss school funding and property tax reform.

Just joking. Back in 1987, Schwarzenegger and Ventura were action movie heroes. In *Predator* the men shoot a variety of weapons, including an M-134 7.62mm minigun and an M-79 grenade launcher.

Now write down a list of speaking tasks that you don't do, that non-stutterers don't think twice about doing. Let's say that you're afraid to leave voicemails on answering machines. Write down all the speech therapy tools you can use in this situation. Imagine yourself as Schwarzenegger and Ventura making a list of weapons to bring. But instead of arming yourself with a minigun and a grenade launcher, your weapons for voicemail could include:

- Practicing your message before you call.
- Fluency skills, such as slow speech with stretched vowels, relaxing your breathing, or relaxing your vocal folds.
- Using a DAF/FAF anti-stuttering device.

- A hierarchy of stress, beginning with calling your own answering machine, then calling your speech-language pathologist's answering machine, then calling a friend's answering machine, then calling a business's answering machine (e.g., calling restaurants before they open asking if they have banquet facilities), and finally calling that attractive person's voicemail.

Don't stop listing your arsenal until you look at the list and laugh at how you'll blow away that poor little voicemail. Then think of one more weapon to add to your list. You're ready when you're confident that you won't stutter.

Let's say that your message is, "You're the most wonderful person I've ever met. I can't wait to see you again." Using all of your fluency weapons, pick up the phone and call your own answering machine. Check your messages. Pretty good, huh?

Now call yourself again. This time, reduce or throw away one of your weapons. If you used one-second stretched syllables on the first call, call yourself using half-second stretch. Then go to quarter-second "slow normal" speech.

If you used an anti-stuttering device on the first call, don't use the device for your next call.

If you practiced the message on the first call, say something spontaneous on your next call.

Step by step, throw away your weapons, until you can call your own voicemail fluently, without effort or fear.

OK, if you're a non-violent person, think of this as a multifactorial approach to stuttering therapy. Instead of relying on one fluency skill, take one item from the auditory processing category (page 11), e.g., an anti-stuttering device; one item from the speech motor control category, e.g., relaxed vocal folds (page 28); one item from the stress control category, e.g., using a hierarchy of stress (page 89); one item from the neurotransmitters category (page 100), e.g., medication, etc. Don't select all your fluency skills from one category, e.g., gentle onsets, diaphragmatic breathing, relaxed vocal folds, etc.

Make a Stress Hierarchy

Now take a step up the stress hierarchy. Call your speech-language pathologist and leave a message. (If you're not in speech therapy, call a friend or relative.) Begin with your full arsenal of fluency weapons, then call back, using fewer fluency weapons. Then work your way up your stress hierarchy. If you feel any twinge of fear on a call, take a step back until you feel confident again.

Approaching feared speaking situations can be like fighting a grizzly bear armed only with a pocket knife. Scary speaking situations combine to look like a ten-foot-tall bear. Most speech therapy programs give you only one weapon.

Divide your general fear of speaking into specific fears. The giant bear becomes many small bears. Now create a stress hierarchy, with a small bear on one end, and a bunny rabbit on the other end. And instead of having one weapon, you now have a variety of fluency skills.

Now you're armed like Arnold Schwarzenegger, you're hunting bunny rabbits, and you're in a pet shop before Easter. Armed to the teeth with speech therapy skills, there's no possibility of stuttering in your feared situation. Heck, it isn't even a feared situation anymore!

You now see why this chapter follows the auditory processing chapter (page 11) and the speech motor learning and control chapter (page 28). The previous chapters gave you many weapons for your fluency arsenal. Now that you have many fluency skills you have no reason to fear speaking situations. Work your way down your list of feared speaking situations until you have no more speech-related fears and anxieties than an average non-stutterer.

Further Reducing Fears and Anxieties

When you run out of speech-related fears and anxieties that non-stutterers aren't scared of, list of speaking situations that scare non-stutterers. Remember when I said that your speech can be better than non-stutterers? When you're ready, move on to these areas:

- Go up to strangers at parties. Say that your speech therapist wants you to talk to strangers and ask if you can talk to this person. If you have an anti-stuttering device, ask if it's OK to use it. No one is going to say no. I met one of my ex-girlfriends this way.

- Join Toastmasters International to learn public speaking.

- Sign up for a beginning acting class at a university or community theater. Acting classes are the most fun you've had since sixth grade.

- Put together some funny stories and perform stand-up comedy on amateur night at a nightclub.

- Sign up for voice lessons. Amaze people by singing at social occasions.

- Learn a foreign language. Talk to cab drivers in their native language.

Stress Is the Absence of Choices

We experience stress when our plans are thwarted. We try to reach a goal, and some little thing stops us. For stutterers, that little thing often is an inability to communicate.

For example, you go to a fast-food restaurant to buy a cheeseburger. You can see the cheeseburgers behind the counter. You can smell the cheeseburgers. You even have correct change in your hand. All you have to do is say, "Cheeseburger"—but stuttering stops you.

Instead of thinking of stress as thwarted plans, think about your choices. You could point at the cheeseburgers. You could write "cheeseburger" on a note. You always have choices.

If you focus only on reaching your goal, you miss opportunities that may be better than your goal. For example, you miss the salmon pesto salad the restaurant just added to the menu.

Or you pantomime "cheeseburger" as if you were playing charades. You feel ridiculous, and people in the line laugh at you. Then a movie producer offers you a million dollars to star in his new "stupid and stupider" movie.

OK, that's unlikely. Just realize that you always have choices. As you imagine your choices, you'll feel your stress going away. Your insurmountable problem now looks like a variety of choices (see the section "Personal Construct Therapy," page 95).

Use a Partner to Center Your Emotions

When you feel stressed, find a partner who expresses the opposite emotion.

For example, you're fired from your job. You come home feeling like a failure and that you'll never succeed. You don't want a partner who agrees with you.

Instead, you want a partner who'll tell you that you're smart and hardworking, and you'll soon find a better job.

Picture your emotions like a car with a manual transmission. To shift from one gear to another gear, you have to shift through neutral. Similarly, to shift from feeling stressed to another emotion, first seek your emotional center.

Reduce Your Child's Stress

No studies have tested whether reducing stress affects children's stuttering. But you can try and observe whether this helps your child's speech.

Don't demand that your child confess guilt (fear of punishment). When your child experiences overwhelming emotions, e.g., is afraid to do something, don't demand that your child explain why he or she feels overwhelmed. Emotions are in a deeper, older brain area. Language is a higher, new brain function. An emotionally overwhelmed child may be unable to speak.

Don't insist that your child talk in an unfamiliar situation, e.g., at a new day care center. Situations that feel comfortable to you may be stressful to your child. Try to see stress from your child's point of view.

Reduce Your Listener's Stress

Stuttering is a rare disorder. Many people have never met a stutterer. I've had listeners ask if I was having a medical emergency, or ask if I was cold (apparently I looked like I was shivering). I have no doubt that other listeners thought that I was mentally retarded or psychotic, perhaps dangerous. Reduce their fears by saying that you stutter.

Some listeners think that they did something to make you stutter. Other listeners wish there were something they could do to help you. Tell them that you stutter. If they have any questions about stuttering, they'll ask you.

Make a joke about stuttering (see page 115). Or put stuttering on your business card, perhaps describing you as chapter leader of your local stuttering support group.

Tell listeners that you're using speech therapy skills. Ask if your fluency skills sound weird, then do what your speech-language pathologist wants you to do (e.g., breathe with your diaphragm, relax your vocal folds, slow down your speaking rate). Ask if your stuttering therapy speech sounds better than your stuttering.

Ask the listener to remind you when you miss a speech motor control target (see page 64).

Lastly, if you use an anti-stuttering device (see page 12), show it to your listener and ask if she minds if you use it. This is perhaps the best way to tell listeners that you stutter. Listeners invariably ask questions about the devices. In contrast, listeners rarely ask questions about speech therapy, e.g., vocal fold relaxation isn't of great interest to the general population. But everyone wants to know how anti-stuttering devices work. Suggest that the listener try on the device, and adjust it to make the listener stutter (by maximizing the delay, or moving the pitch shift up and down). When I do this, other people come over to see what's making their friend trip over his or her words. They give me positive feedback about my stuttering, laugh at their own failure to talk, and experience for a few minutes what it feels like to stutter.

Alternative Ways to Reduce Stress

If stuttering is the only way you know to reduce stress, you'll always stutter in stressful situations. Instead, learn alternative ways to reduce stress. Take a stress reduction class. Read books about handling stress.

One of the best ways to reduce stress is to relax your breathing. Stress reduction classes teach this. Or take a meditation or yoga class. Relaxed breathing not only reduces stress, it helps stutterers talk fluently.

Look for Stuttering-Reducers

A stutterer reads a projected PowerPoint presentation aloud to an audience. He scans the slides for feared words. Sure enough, there's a p-word. And an s-word! He consults the prodigious thesaurus in his brain, looking for words he can substitute. But the audience is reading the slides on the screen. Will they think he's illiterate if he substitutes or skips words? But what if he blocks and the audience discovers that he stutters! What a dilemma!

He's looking for stuttering-increasers, i.e., ways to stutter. And, sure enough, stuttering-increasers—difficult sounds, feared words, judgmental listeners—abound, if you know where to find them.

Imagine another stutterer, also reading aloud to an audience. Instead of looking for stuttering-increasers, she looks for stuttering-reducers:

- With her text prepared for her, she can focus on using her speech therapy skills instead of thinking about what she's saying.

- She can pretend to be a robot reading machine. The robot has no emotions, it just sees words, moves its mouth, and words come out.

- She can wear an anti-stuttering device and the audience will think it's a microphone for the PA system.

- When she introduces herself she can say that she stutters. Audiences love presentations that start with a joke, so she could start with a joke about her stuttering (page 115).

Increasing or Decreasing Stress in Therapy

Stuttering therapy typically begins with a stutterer learning closed-loop speech motor control in a low-stress environment, e.g., chatting with the speech-language pathologist, or alone practicing word lists.

The stutterer gradually moves from closed-loop speech motor control to open-loop speech motor control. When he achieves fluent open-loop speech motor control, the speech-language pathologist takes him to a shopping mall for "transfer" practice. Then they're finished with speech therapy and he's on his own.

The result is fluent open-loop speech in low-stress environments, and relapse to open-loop stuttering in high-stress environments. The relapse shakes the stutterer's self-confidence. Or the stress de-myelinates (weakens) fluent speech motor programs. A single high-stress, dysfluent experience might destroy weeks of low-stress practice.

The stutterer then gets into a vicious cycle of stress and relapse leading to more stress and more relapse.

A better plan would be to train a stutterer to recognize stressful situations, and consciously switch to closed-loop speech motor control (i.e., very slow speech, page 33) in high-stress environments. When he feels his stress diminishing he can switch to open-loop speech motor control (i.e., normal-sounding speech).

For example, I used to meet strangers and say, "My speech-language pathologist wants me to talk to strangers. May I talk to you?" I would then use slow closed-loop speech motor control. After we had a friendly conversation going and my fears and anxieties diminished, I'd use the "slow-normal" speaking rate that mixes open- and closed-loop speech motor control.

In other words, with traditional therapy the stutterer switches between stuttering and fluent speech, as situations change between high-stress and low-stress. Instead, I switched between closed-loop and open-loop speech motor control, as stress changed. The result was that I constantly myelinated (strengthened) the fluent speech motor programs in my brain. I also strengthened my brain's connection between stressful situations and closed-loop speech motor control. Switching to closed-loop speech motor control in a stressful situation should be as habitual as counting to ten before punching someone.

Some severe stutterers may be unable to produce even two-second stretch closed-loop speech motor control in stressful situations. In other words, their fluent speech completely breaks down under stress. So use the *Predator* approach (page 87).

Or you might object that closed-loop speech motor control sounds "weird," and stressful situations are where you most want to sound normal. When I said to strangers, "My speech-language pathologist wants me to talk to strangers…" no one ever refused. Most people then asked me questions about stuttering therapy. As long as the stutterer tells listeners that he is using special "speech therapy speech," sounding "weird" isn't an issue.

Personal Construct Therapy: You Always Have Choices

> No one needs to be completely hemmed in by circum-stances; no one needs to be the victim of his biography.[61]
> — George Kelly, *The Psychology of Personal Constructs*
> (1955)

In every situation, you always have a choice of how to react. This insight is the basis of *personal construct therapy* (PCT). The goal of PCT is to develop awareness of your choices in every situation. The antithesis is to react the same way to all stressful situations.

If you make the same speech choices in high-stress situations, no amount of practice in a low-stress speech clinic will change your speech. For example, if you always substitute words "when the going gets tough," you're not going to use gentle onsets in a difficult situations, even after practicing 5,000 gentle onsets in the speech clinic.

To develop awareness of your choices, describe a situation in which you stuttered. Imagine different ways you could have responded to the situation.

Role-play the scene with your speech-languge pathologist or in your support group. When someone sees a choice that hasn't been played, switch roles, for that person to play the new choice. For example, the situation is answering the telephone at work. One person pretends to be a caller, and the other pretends to be the employee answering at Pasquale's Pizza. The employee uses slow speech. But another choice might be to switch to voiced consonants (page 48), i.e., answering the phone *Basdahllee's Bizza.* You should be able to think of a half-dozen other possibilities. Role play each choice and see what feels best.

Slow Down by Not Interrupting

Conscious choice requires slow reactions. In a fast reaction to environmental stimuli, your brain will select the most myelinated (habitual) open-loop motor program (page 30). Interrupting people, or responding quickly in a conversation, is a fast reaction.

Let people finish their sentences. Wait two seconds. Then start talking. Your fluency will improve.

Verbal Aikido

Aikido is a Japanese martial art. Combatants focus not on punching or kicking opponents, but rather on using the opponent's own energy to gain control of the opponent or to throw the opponent away from you.[62]

Verbal aikido is the art of not arguing, but instead agreeing with someone who is verbally attacking you. You help the assailant attack you, until—surprise—he realizes that he's just been made to look like a fool.

For example, a middle-aged, overweight woman owned a chain of women-only health clubs. Middle-aged, overweight women could work out in these health clubs without feeling intimidated by young male bodybuilders.

A "shock jock" radio host invited the health club owner onto his show. He described her physical appearance, then asked why anyone would want to work out at a health club owned by a fat, ugly old lady.

She responded, "So we don't have to work out with boorish meatheads like you."

This silenced the radio host long enough for her to say that overweight, middle-aged ladies have to exercise too, and the "shock jock" was a perfect example of the men she didn't want to have to be around when she exercised.

The example of the parents responding to their teenagers' four-letter words (page 126) is another example of verbal aikido.

Use verbal aikido to turn around the stress. For example, a highway patrol officer pulls you over for speeding. Instead of trying to hide your stuttering, you make a joke: "I stutter, so I'm not going to try to talk you out of giving me a ticket." Maybe this will put the officer in a good mood and let you go with a warning.

Changing Self-Descriptions

Many stutterers improve their speech, yet continue to believe that their speech is worse than non-stutterers. Graduates of fluency shaping therapy programs sometimes have beautiful, clear speech that is easier and more pleasant to listen to than non-stutterers' speech. Yet they continue to believe that they can't do certain things, such as public speaking.[63]

In contrast, stutterers who improve their speech attitudes have better speech a year after completing therapy, as compared to stutterers who maintain poor attitudes.[64]

Write a description of yourself now, and who you expect to be in five years. What items are opposite in the two descriptions? E.g., now you're now single, but in five years you hope to be married.

Write a description of yourself as a stutterer, and then who you'd be if you didn't stutter. E.g., assertive vs. shy, or popular vs. lonely. These descriptions are your *personal constructs*.

Work on changing your personal constructs. Again, imagine specific situations for each personal construct. For example, if you wrote that you'd be assertive instead of shy, describe a recent situation in which you weren't assertive. Now role-play the scene with your speech-language pathologist or your support group. Imagine different ways to react in the situation and switch roles.

"Who Would I Be If I Didn't Stutter?"

This is a favorite conversation topic at stuttering support groups. People initially say, "I'd be more successful at work" or "I'd be more assertive with my husband and family." They first think their lives would be better without stuttering.

After fifteen minutes, people start saying, "If I didn't stutter, I'd be less compassionate," or "I would never have developed my musical talent." People realize that they chose a career in a "helping profession" (e.g., nursing or teaching), or they developed non-verbal skills, such as athletics or painting, because they stutter. They realize *positive* aspects of stuttering. They see that stuttering can be a gift.

In contrast, a stutterer completed a speech therapy program, but refused to speak fluently. He said that his co-workers had listened to his stuttering for 20 years. He asked, "What would they think if I came to work speaking fluently?"

Another stutterer was earning $25,000/year as a computer programmer. His supervisor left, and the company wanted to promote the stutterer. He would receive a salary of $55,000/year. The management position required talking to clients on the telephone. The company offered to pay for speech therapy and an anti-stuttering device. The stutterer refused the promotion, saying that he didn't want to talk to anyone. The company instead hired a less-qualified manager from outside the company.

For these stutterers, the psychological issues surrounding stuttering are more disabling than their disfluencies.

Change Your Lifestyle

As your improve your fluency, ask your supervisor for tasks that require talking. Participate in social activities that involve talking.

Training a new motor skill requires about three million repetitions (page 68). To say three million words, you must talk at least four hours a day for at least six months.

Take an acting class. Take singing lessons. You'll have fun, and meet new people. You'll get over your speech-related fears.

You'll find some things other people can easily do that you can't, but you'll also find things you can easily do that other people can't. For example, I took a public speaking course. I was able to project my voice, when other students are afraid to raise their voices. I was able to switch emotions (anger, sadness) easily and convincingly, when other students couldn't. On the other hand, there were simple presentations where you couldn't understand a word I said.

Volunteer to read to blind or elderly individuals. Volunteer at a hospital directing visitors where to go. Volunteer with your public radio station answering pledge week calls.

Or moonlight at a job that requires talking. Find a job that requires being charming and friendly.

Join social clubs that requires talking. Put Toastmasters at the top of your list. Members give a series of ten speeches, usually one speech per month. The speeches are four to ten minutes long. Each of the ten speeches teaches you a new skill, such as using gestures and body language, or being persuasive on a controversial topic. Judges always point out things you did well—and award lots of ribbons—as well as ways you can improve. You'll find that even if you stutter severely, you're better than non-stutterers at some aspects of public speaking.

The National Stuttering Association has its own public speaking training program, which is quite different from Toastmasters. Ask for the "Speaking Circles" video.

Anti-Stuttering Medications

The neurotransmitter *dopamine* makes you feel alert, motivated, and mentally acute. When you feel "energy," your brain has plenty of dopamine. Caffeine, cocaine, and amphetamines produce their "buzz" by affecting your brain's dopamine.

A study found that three genes that affect dopamine correlate with five disorders: attention deficit hyperactivity disorder (ADHD), Tourette's syndrome, stuttering, obsessive-compulsive disorder (OCD), and tics.[65] All five disorders result in undesirable behaviors that manifest when the person experiences stress but not when the person is relaxed. Trying to control the behavior or movement makes it worse and more difficult to control. (Read the Wikipedia article about Tourette's. Or invite a Tourette's support group to meet with your stuttering support group.)

Dopamine antagonist medications reduce stuttering. However, these medications have side effects, and the long-term effects are unknown. Rather than taking medication indefinitely, it may be better for a severe adult stutterer to combine medication with other stuttering therapy and reduce his dosage as his fluency improves, until he no longer needs the medication.

If you suspect that your child's medication contributes to his or her stuttering—especially if your child is on several medications—I suggest that you consult a pharmacist who specializes in stuttering and medications, such as Richard Harkness (http://members.aol.com/rharkn/).

"Good Days, Bad Days"—and the Anti-Stuttering Diet
Stutterers have "good days"—with less stuttering—and "bad days"—when they can't get a word out. The "good days/bad days" syndrome may be due to varying levels of neurotransmitters.

Dopamine is affected by several factors, including diet. Dopamine is produced from the amino acids phenylalanine and tyrosine. Both amino acids are components of protein. Meat sources of protein have more tyrosine than plant sources of protein. The exception is wheat germ, which is high in tyrosine. The foods highest in phenylalanine are soy and fish.

A vegetarian, wheat-free, low-protein diet should lower dopamine levels. I tried this. I stuttered less, but felt sluggish and depressed. I'd rather eat protein, feel mentally alert, and stutter.

In *The Edge Effect* (2005; ISBN 1-4027-2247-8), psychiatrist Eric Braverman presents the four neurotransmitters (dopamine, acetylcholine, GABA, and serotonin) and suggests that health and well-being relates to balancing the four via diet, supplements, and/or medication. The book includes a questionnaire that shows which of your neurotransmitters are higher or lower (no one is perfectly balanced) and if any are out of normal range. My score indicated that dopamine was my lowest neurotransmitter and acetylcholine was my highest, but all were within normal range. If this is true, then lowering my dopamine wouldn't make sense. But if your score showed high dopamine, than maybe diet, supplements, and/or medications are something you should look into. If you do the questionnaire, e-mail me the results. It'll be interesting to see if stutterers are on average high or low on dopamine.

Dopamine Antagonists

Dopamine antagonists reduce dopamine activity. In general, these medications reduce stuttering.

Haldol

Haloperidol (Haldol) is an old dopamine antagonist. It was the first medication to reduce stuttering in two clinical trials.

The side effects can be severe. A stutterer took it for several days, then one night found his head rotating slowly back and forth 180 degrees—and there was nothing he could do to stop it! The effect on his speech had been minimal, so he stopped taking the medication.

Risperdal

Newer medications more narrowly target certain dopamine receptors. The dopamine D_2-receptor antagonist risperidone (Risperdal) reduces stuttering about 50%.[66] Like other stuttering therapies, the drug is most effective in low-stress situations, and least effective in high-stress situations.

The drug is FDA-approved only for short-term (6-8 week) treatment of schizophrenia. Side effects include insomnia, agitation, anxiety, somnolence, extrapyramidal nervous system disorders, headaches, dizziness, constipation, rhinitis (a breathing disorder), rashes, tachycardia (a heart disorder), and breast growth in men and women (due to increased levels of the hormone prolactin), and neuroleptic malignant syndrome (potentially fatal).

A stutterer tried Risperdal, and couldn't leave his house due to severe anxiety.

Another male stutterer wrote, "I used Risperdal for about 6 months. It had a marginal (if any) effect on the intensity of my stutter. I had to discontinue its use due to hormonal side-effects (my right breast started to grow)."

Zyprexa

Olanzapine (Zyprexa) reduces stuttering on average 33%.[67] Side effects are mostly limited to slight weight gain and drowsiness.[68]

Other Dopamine Antagonists

Pimozide[69] and Tiapride[70] are other dopamine antagonists that have been reported to help stutterers.

Dopamine Agonists

Dopamine agonist medications increase dopamine activity (the opposite of dopamine antagonists). Increasing dopamine should increase stuttering. However, no published research has explored the effects of dopamine agonists on stuttering. Based on anecdotal reports, stutterers may want to consider avoiding dopamine agonists, including caffeine, cocaine, and amphetamines.

Ritalin

Ritalin is a dopamine agonist. A speech pathologist asked on the Internet:

> I'm treating an 8-year-old diagnosed ADHD and who suddenly began stuttering (advanced core and secondary behaviors) without any prior history of dysfluency, as a side effect of the medication Ritalin. He's had a whole neuro work-up which revealed nothing.

Another speech pathologist responded that many of the children he treated for stuttering were on Ritalin for ADHD.

Pharmacist Richard Harkness advises against Ritalin for children who stutter:

> Ritalin increases dopaminergic neurotransmission and is contraindicated for use in those with Tourette's disorder. Ritalin has also, in rare cases, brought on symptoms of Tourette's disorder. Tourette's disorder has been likened to stuttering in that it involves a flaw in dopaminergic neurotransmission.

Other Neurotransmitters

Clinical trials are underway for what could be the first FDA-approved anti-stuttering medications. Pagoclone is a gamma amino butyric acid (GABA) selective receptor modulator.[71]

Dopamine and acetylcholine tend to work in balance in some disorders. An increase in one tends to decrease the other. It's possible that stuttering results from too little acetylcholine as well as too much dopamine, and that dopamine antagonsts also act as acetylcholine agonists when they affect stuttering.[72]

Antidepressants Increase Stuttering

Some antidepressant medications boost dopamine. These medications include the selective serotonin reuptake inhibitor (SSRI) class, which includes Prozac and Zoloft. These medications have increased stuttering in stutterers. In a few cases, these drugs caused non-stutterers to stutter.

Stutterers taking SSRI anti-depressants report feeling less depression, but their increased stuttering makes them feel worse:

> I was sitting in the hallway, in the dark. I had been crying and hitting my head on the wall, screaming to God, why me? I hated my stuttering and I suppose hated myself as well. From that point on it was as if when I remembered that incident all the feelings came back to me and wouldn't leave. Those angry, hurt, frustrating feelings from so long ago wouldn't go away. I was hiding my feelings from everyone around me, pretending to be super mom and super wife. I decided to seek professional help.
>
> We decided that I would try Wellbutrin. As my doctor put it, kill two birds with one stone, since Wellbutrin is also prescribed to help you quit smoking. The first week I felt like I had so much anxiety that I could explode. The second week I noticed my stuttering getting worse. By the third week the controls that I had learned in speech therapy were virtually unusable. It was so frustrating to not be able to control my stuttering at all. Needless to say we all agreed to flush the Wellbutrin and never go back on anything like that.
>
> Prozac, Trazadone and Effexor did not effect my speech at all.[73]

Another stutterer wrote:

> I have tried 3 antidepressants: Prozac, Wellbutrin, and Zoloft. All increased my stuttering noticeably. The antidepressants that I have tried make me more able to get out of bed in the morning and restore my "get up and go"; however, they have caused me to go from being a

person with a barely noticeable stutter to a more pro-
nounced stutter.

I went in to my psychiatrist yesterday and explained
that the current antidepressant is making my stutter
signficantly worse. However, in the 10 minutes we talked
I was practically perfectly fluent. He then concludes that
obviously "it's not that unmanageable."

He prescribed 10mg Propanolol to take before I have
to be in a difficult speaking presentation. It is supposed
to "reduce performance anxiety." I don't feel like I have
a tremendous amount of performance anxiety; stuttering
just isn't very fun. I think he doesn't believe me about
the severity of the stuttering.

Other Medications

Botulinum Toxin

Botox, the toxin in botulism, has been injected into stutterers'
vocal folds. The toxin partially paralyzes your vocal folds so you
can't get into hard blocks. You also can't talk loudly or forcefully.
The toxin reduces stuttering somewhat. It wears off in a few
months, and you get a second shot. The second shot reduces
stuttering less than the first. By the third shot, the toxin usually has
no effect on stuttering.

Tranquilizers

Some doctors prescribe tranquilizers to stutterers on the erroneous
belief that nervousness causes stuttering.

A psychiatrist had some pills he thought might help.
Einer was to take one per day during the week remain-
ing before the great day, and one extra big super pill on
the morning of the wedding. The pills made him feel
somewhat relaxed but had no noticeable effect on his
speech. The wedding arrived, Einer took his super pill,
and went off to London on the train to meet his relatives
who had come for the ceremony.

An hour before the wedding Einer had still not returned. I kept the smiling calm that I had learned to assume in the face of all our difficulties and began dressing. Half an hour later I stood in white satin complete with veil and bouquet, looking out of the bedroom window towards the railway station, wondering what could have happened and preparing myself mentally for a last minute cancellation of the wedding. Had he thrown himself under a train, unable to continue life as a stutterer? Had he run back to Canada as a supreme act of avoidance? The minutes ticked by. Finally another train pulled in, and up the hill walked Einer, a lazy smile on his face, apparently unaware of the panic that he had caused. He had forgotten to take pencil and paper and so was unable to ask for guidance and had become hopelessly lost. However, the super pill had kept him smiling. I am glad to say that thanks to the kindly vicar in reading along with Einer, the wedding vows were the first and only fluent words my family heard Einer speak that summer.[74]

In general, tranquilizers have "more effect on the complexity or severity of the [stuttered] blocks than on their frequency."[75]

Alcohol

No researchers have studied the effects of alcohol on stuttering. (Finding volunteers wouldn't be a problem at most universities!) Anecdotally, alcohol reduces stutterers' fears and anxieties (e.g., about talking to persons of the opposite sex) and so reduces stuttering. But alcohol reduces one's ability to use therapy techniques, and so increases stuttering.

Psychological Issues

In 1928, a Freudian psychologist advanced a theory that stuttering was an attempt to satisfy unresolved oral-erotic needs.[76] If this were true, there would stuttering phone sex lines. Imagine finding ads in the back of *Playboy* magazine with scantily dressed women saying, "Call me! I stutter!"

A 1939 personality test study found that stutterers were more neurotic, more introverted, less dominant, less self-confident, and less sociable than non-stutterers.[77] Examination of the personality test found sixteen speech-related questions, including "If you are dining out do you prefer someone else to order dinner for you?" The psychologists had interpreted stutterers' reluctance to order in restaurants as evidence of neuroses, rather than as difficulty talking.

A 1952 study of hostility and aggression found stutterers more likely to turn hostility inward. A 1953 study found the opposite.[78]

Other psychological studies found no difference between stutterers and non-stutterers for self-concept, levels of aspiration, body images, role perception, handwriting, social maturity, birth order, exaggerated fears, sleep disturbances, hyperactivity, temper tantrums, thumb sucking, and nail biting.[79]

Stutterers are, on average, psychologically normal, except for fears and anxieties around talking. We generally have the same speech-related fears and anxieties as non-stutterers, such as fear of talking to strangers and fear of speaking to an audience, but these fears are greater in stutterers.

Locus of Control

Have you joined one of the stuttering support e-mail lists? I'll save you the effort of reading hundreds of e-mails. There are only two e-mails on the support lists. The first says:

> I don't have a job because I'm afraid co-workers will discover that I stutter. I don't have a girlfriend because I've never asked a woman out on a date. My friends cross the street to avoid me when they see me coming. I'm 47 years old and I live with my parents. Stuttering has made me a miserable wretch. Why isn't there a cure for stuttering? I spend all day hoping that doctors will find a cure.

The other e-mail says:

> Hang in there! You can do it! Have faith! We're all behind you, and in the same boat!

OK, there are a few other e-mails. Every week there's one that says:

> I just heard about acupuncture (hypnosis, Reiki, St. John's Wort, primal scream therapy, electroshock, trepanation, leeches). My cousin's friend's brother-in-law tried it for ingrown toenails and said it was a miracle! Has anyone tried it for stuttering? I'll bet it'll cure me!

Then there's the guy who's discovered the cure for stuttering, and responds to every e-mail with a six-page description of his psycho-neuro-proctological theory of and treatment for stuttering.

On page 9 I referenced a study suggesting that about two million American adults stutter, and presented facts suggesting that only about 20,000 adult stutterers have sought treatment. Is it possible that 99% of adult stutterers never seek treatment? Are 99% of adult stutterers miserable wretches who never leave home?

Locus of control is associated with assignment of causality of a given condition. A person with an *internal locus of control* sees stuttering, and stuttering therapy, as something that he does. A person with an *external locus of control* sees stuttering as something that happens to him, and therapy as something that a speech-language pathologist does to him.

A study found that internal vs. external locus of control did *not* predict fluency two years after completing a stuttering therapy program.[80] In other words, an individual who says, "I can beat stuttering if I try hard harder" doesn't become more fluent than a person who believes that "achieving fluency...is nearly impossible" and "stuttering is a physical impediment for which little can be done."[81] Locus of control alone isn't a factor in stuttering.

However, that study only looked at one stuttering therapy program. Possibly different stuttering treatments are more effective for persons with internal vs. external loci of control.

If you have an external locus of control, you might get better results with anti-stuttering medications or with anti-stuttering devices set for a normal speaking rate—treatments that do things to you.

If you have an internal locus of control, you might get better results from fluency shaping therapy, anti-stuttering devices set to assist fluency shaping therapy, and working on handling stress better—treatments that you do for yourself.

Internal Locus of Control Pitfalls

If you say, "I've been to stuttering therapy, I just have to remember to use my therapy skills" then you have an internal locus of control, and you're headed for a trap.

An internal locus of control can make you blind to people who could help you, e.g., you refuse to join a stuttering support group.

An internal locus of control can make you blind to other stuttering treatments, e.g., your state offers to give you a free anti-stuttering telephone.

External Locus of Control Pitfalls

Consider why crazy weight loss diets attract customers. People try the "pizza and ice cream" diet, it doesn't work, and then they can say that they tried to lose weight but the diet didn't work. There-fore no diet, exercise plan, or anything else will ever work. Therefore they have an excuse to be overweight. These people chose the "pizza and ice cream" diet instead of the salads and running ten miles a day diet. They chose a fad diet because they knew it wouldn't work.

Similarly, if you have an external locus of control, go to speech therapy, and it doesn't work, you may conclude that no stuttering treatment works.

Locus of Control Is Not Motivation

It may look like an internal locus of control is the same as motiva-tion, and individuals with external loci of control are lazy bums. But go to a National Stuttering Association convention and you'll meet hundreds of motivated, external locus of control stutterers. These people work hard to host support groups, organize events for stutterers, and write zillions of e-mails on e-mail lists.

Let's look at some workshops offered at the 2006 National Stut-tering Association annual convention: "Flying with Attitude," "Building Self-Confidence," "Getting to the Bottom of Your Fears," "Coping with Stuttering in a Social World," "Stepping Out of Our Comfort Zone," and a workshop that demonstrated how to

> "switch gears" to a self-approving position by giving oneself credit for any degree of progress made or trying to be made rather than yielding to all the familiar nega-tive and self-defeating thoughts which tend to overwhelm any degree of success.[82]

The convention also had two workshops about anti-stuttering devices, a speech from a psychiatrist with expertise in anti-stuttering medications, and a talk about genetic research. But mostly the convention was about not feeling bad about yourself in environments and situations beyond your control. In other words, the convention was for people with external loci of control.

Denial

I had a neighbor with schizophrenia. Since its onset in his twenties (he was in his forties the last time I saw him), he'd lost his job as a chemical engineer and now worked as a minimum wage security guard. He'd never asked a woman out on a date since the voices in his head started. He rented a room in the house next door to where I lived. He had no friends other than me.

Like 40% of people with schizophrenia, he denied that he had the disorder. He was convinced that when he'd gone for a root canal, the dentist had inserted a radio receiver in his tooth, and now the CIA was broadcasting voices into his head.

My neighbor enjoyed reading French and Italian newspapers at a university library. He'd take the newspapers to the basement where no one would hear him repeating obscenities to annoy the CIA agents listening to his thoughts. One day, security guards asked him to leave. To get away from them he ran into traffic in a busy street. He wasn't allowed in the library after that.

Consider what would have happened if he'd told a librarian that he had a mental illness that made him talk to himself, and asked if there was somewhere he could read the newspapers without disturbing anyone. The librarian would have unlocked a conference room for him to use.

Denying that he had schizophrenia took effort. His life would have been simpler if he admitted that he had the disorder. *If you put more effort into denying that you have a disorder than the treatment would demand, then you have a denial problem.*

He asked me whether I thought he was crazy. I said, "You're crazy if you deny that you have a mental illness. If you admit it, then you're not crazy."

Denial in Stuttering

Again you might be tempted to think of people who are in denial as lazy bums, but look again. My neighbor worked hard, almost every minute of the day, to refuse to believe that he had schizophrenia.

Stutterers who are in denial work harder than stutterers who are open about their stuttering. For example, many stutterers will spend an hour driving to a store to see if the store has an item, instead of spending two minutes calling the store.

Or saying "the great American pastime" instead of "baseball." That's eight syllables instead of two, and some listeners won't know what you're talking about.

A woman called me, inquiring about my company's anti-stuttering devices. Her husband was a computer software engineer. He'd stopped talking. He'd requested a demotion at work to a position in which he never spoke to anyone. He sat in his cubicle, communicating by e-mail. At home he no longer spoke to his wife or children. He stopped participating in social activities or friend-ships. His wife was considering divorce. But first she was learning everything she could about stuttering, in hopes of finding some-thing that would enable him to speak.

Did this man have a stuttering problem? Or did he have a denial problem? He thought he could make his life easier by not talking. But the effort required to not talk (e.g., an unhappy marriage) outweighed the effort of talking (e.g., to his wife, who already knew and accepted that he stuttered).

The Most Important Aspect of Your Life

Let me tell you about an accountant I had dinner with. He worked for the local government. He kept pen and paper next to his bed because he'd wake up with ideas of how to solve accounting problems at work.

My first thought was, this guy needs a life! He dreams about accounting!

Then I thought, he thinks about accounting 24/7. He must be a good accountant. When I need an accountant I'll hire him.

Until I was 22 and saw myself on video, I was unaware how severely I stuttered. I thought that I had a minor speech problem. I tried to do everything that everyone else does. When I failed at things most people seemed to effortlessly achieve (e.g., finding a job, finding a girlfriend) I didn't realize it was because talking to me was an excruciating experience for listeners. No one told me that. They just avoided me.

When I was 30 I realized that stuttering wasn't something that I could compensate for by excelling at other things. Stuttering affected every aspect of my life. I changed the focus of my life. I thought about stuttering 24/7. I'd wake up with ideas for how to solve speech problems. Speech therapy changed from something I did two hours a week, to what I did all the time.

Whatever you focus on, you can achieve. It may take years of persistence but you will succeed. But you can only think about one thing 24/7. You don't want to spend your life climbing a mountain, get to the top, then see that you climbed the wrong mountain.

Is stuttering the most important aspect of your life? If you're a severe stutterer, as I was, the answer may be yes. Focus on stuttering 24/7. Your speech will improve, and then everything else will fall into place. For example, your speech improves, then your boss gives you a promotion. Then the pretty blonde at the photo store wants to be your girlfriend. It happened to me, and it'll happen to you. Read more stories like this in the chapter "Famous People Who Stutter" (page 139).

But if you're a mild stutterer, stuttering might be the wrong mountain for you to climb. You might be focusing your energy on stuttering, when listeners don't care whether you stutter. They might even like hearing you stutter mildly. Your life isn't going to change until you focus your energy elsewhere.

Freedom to Speak—Badly

I found this in the book *How to Learn Any Language*:

> Americans, however, hold one high card that too frequently goes unplayed. We're gregarious. We're extroverts. Some say it contemptuously. Some say it admiringly. But those who know us best agree that we

> Americans are the only people in the world who enjoy speaking another language badly!
>
> Most people in the world are shy, embarrassed, even paralyzed when it comes to letting themselves be heard in languages they speak less than fluently. An American may master a foreign language to the point where he considers himself fluent. A European, however, who speaks a language equally well and no better will often deny he speaks it at all! [83]

Are you an American—happy to talk even when your speech isn't good? Or are you a European—"shy, embarrassed, even paralyzed" when you can't speak fluently?

The First Amendment to our Constitution is freedom of *speech*. The Founding Fathers believed that talking is the most basic human right. Generations of Americans have fought for that right. Stick an American flag pin in your lapel and go out and speak—badly, if you have to.

Change Your Lifestyle to Talk More

Ask your supervisor to give you work requiring talking. This could be talking to customers, or calling suppliers, or training other employees.

Or change careers to a job that requires talking. A man bought an anti-stuttering device, quit his job as a back room accountant at a bank, then worked at the Chicago Board of Trade, yelling orders to buy and sell soybean futures. Now he's a law school professor.

Or find a volunteer service requiring talking. Hospitals have information booths where volunteers direct visitors to their floors. Public television stations need volunteers to answer the phones during pledge drives.

Political groups need canvassers to collect signatures on petitions. Pick a cause you believe in. Imagine yourself standing on a busy street corner, talking to passerby about an important issue. Can you picture anything more American?

Complimenting People

Here's another way to make the world a better place. Make eye contact, smile, and then compliment a person.

Don't limit this to attractive, single persons. Make everyone you meet feel good about themselves. Compliment old men, women pushing strollers in the park, the person behind you in the supermarket line, and your in-laws.

- Compliment the person's smile. Then smile. This will make the person smile. Add a little joke such as, "Give my compliments to your orthodontist."

- Compliment the person's eyes. This reminds you to make eye contact. Look into the person's eyes long enough to mentally note his or her eye color. A friend broke up with her boyfriend when, wearing sunglasses, she asked him what color her eyes were. He didn't know.

- Compliment the person's name. This helps you remember the person's name. Associate the person's name with an interesting fact, e.g., ask how his or her name is spelled (e.g., Rebecca vs. Rebekah), the ethnic origin, or the meaning of the name. Read a history of your area to learn the names of local heroes and historical figures.

- Compare the person to a celebrity. (A friend writing a personal ad asked if she looked like Natalie Merchant or Neve Campbell. I replied that she reminded me more of a young Tommy Lee Jones.)

- Listen for extraordinary things people have done, then reflect this back to them. Everyone thinks that their lives are ordinary. For example, a man who flies jet fighters thinks of himself as an ordinary fighter pilot.

Tell Stuttering Jokes

Here's a few of my favorite stuttering jokes:

A stutterer goes away to a two-week intensive speech therapy course on the East Coast. When he returns, his friends ask how it went.

The stutterer pauses, takes a deep breath, and slowly says, "Peter Piper picked a peck of pickled peppers."

His friends are amazed. "You said that completely fluently!" they say.

The stutterer says, "Y-y-yeah b-b-but it's, it's h-h-hard t-t-to w-w-work th-that in-t-to a, a c-c-conversation."

It was his first time at skydiving class, and the young man was thrilled.

"What you have to do," said the instructor, "is jump, count to ten, then pull the ripcord."

The young man was so excited that he really wasn't paying too close attention. He turned to the instructor and said, "P-p-p-p-pardon m-m-m-me, wh-wh-wh-wh-what w-w-w-was th-th-th-th-that n-n-n-n-number ag-ag-again?"

"Two," the instructor replied.

An old man on a flight to Rome got talking to the fellow seated beside him and couldn't help noticing he had one heck of a stutter. He was even more astonished when his new acquaintance told him, with difficulty, that he was going for an audition as an announcer for Radio Vatican.

"How do you rate your chances?" asked the old man.

"Na, na, na, not too good," he replied. "They will pa, pa, probably g, g, give the job job t, t, to some ba, bloody Catholic!"

Inward vs. Outward Anger

Stuttering, like any frustrating experience, causes anger. Some individuals direct these feelings inward (i.e., they hate themselves). This leads to a vicious cycle or "self-fulfilling prophecy" of failure.

But other stutterers direct these feelings outward. These individuals feel anger at other people. Their relationships at work or socially go poorly, again creating a vicious cycle of failure.

How do you feel when people disrespect you when you stutter? Do you feel anger at yourself for stuttering? Or do you feel anger at the person who treated you poorly?

When you're angry, do you do nothing, but get angrier inside? That's inner-directed self-hatred.

Or do you take action to "send a message" nonverbally—which the other person is certain to misunderstand? I once "sent a message" to my housemates that it was their turn to buy toilet paper. Don't ask me what I did! They didn't get the message. They just got angry back at me. That didn't lead to domestic bliss.

Earlier I suggested that you use slow, stretched syllables when telemarketers call (see page 65). Do you look forward to annoying telemarketers? If so, you direct your anger outward. But if you're afraid to annoy telemarketers, then you direct your anger inward.

If practicing speech therapy with a telemarketer scares you, have your speech-language pathologist pretend to call you. She'll try to sell you slow pitch bats, slow blow fuses, stainless steel slow cookers, and slow jam CDs. If you can't think of anything to say, ask, "How slow are the slow pitch bats?"

Then call her, reversing roles. Convince her that your slow cookers are the slowest, and that no one makes a slower slow jam CD. Practice this until you're willing to practice therapy skills with a telemarketer.

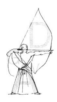

Childhood Stuttering

The average age of stuttering onset is 30 months (two-and-half-years-old).[84] Stuttering rarely begins after age six.

65% of preschoolers who stutter spontaneously recover, in their first two years of stuttering.[85] These children grow up to have normal speech.[86] However, children who stutter longer are less likely to recover without treatment. Only 18% of children who stutter five years recover spontaneously.[87] The peak age of recovery is three and a half years old. By age six, a child is unlikely to recover without speech therapy.

Among preschoolers, boys who stutter outnumber girls who stutter about two to one, or fewer.[88] But more girls recover fluent speech, and more boys don't.[89] By fifth grade the ratio is about four boys who stutter to one girl who stutters. This ratio remains into adulthood.[90]

Some pediatricians tell parents to "wait and see" if a child outgrows stuttering on his own. That advice is wrong. Children who stutter should see a speech-language pathologist as soon as possible. To find a speech-language pathologist for your child, start by calling your school. American schools provide free speech therapy to children as young as three years old.

If your child stutters at two or three, and you get the child into speech therapy right away, you can expect a full recovery, within months, without relapses. A small nudge will get your child back onto the normal development track.

If your child is in grade school and has stuttered for five years, he or she will need a bigger shove to get back onto the normal development track.

Five Stages of Stuttering Development

At two or three years old, children are quickly developing communication skills. Their brains are growing rapidly. A child's language skills may develop faster than his speech skills. He wants to communicate but can't easily and freely generate speech.

The "conventional wisdom" among stuttering experts is that children move in a series of five stages from normal dysfluencies into stuttering.

Stage One: Normal Disfluency (Ages 2–6)

All children have normal dysfluencies as they learn speech and language. Normal dysfluencies aren't stuttering, and don't need to be treated by a speech-language pathologist.

Normal dysfluencies tend to be single, such as "That my-my ball," or "I want some…uh…juice."

Normal dysfluencies tend to be interjections (sounds or syllables), revisions (of words, phrases, sentences, or story), and whole-word repetitions (not part-word repetitions).

The child doesn't manifest struggle behaviors or visible tension, frustration or embarrassment. The child experiences dysfluencies as if he stumbled while walking, and recovered his balance and continued walking.

Normal dysfluencies occur when the child is planning a long or complex language structure. Brief silent pauses are considered normal. Normal disfluencies also occur under "pragmatic" conditions, such as when directing another person's activity, when concerned about the listener's reaction, and when interrupting or being interrupted.

Normal dysfluencies may occur when the child's language skills exceed his speech motor skills. Or he may be so busy learning to walk or refine other motor skills that his speech skills don't develop rapidly enough.

Changes in the child's environment may also cause temporary normal dysfluencies. This could involve parents' divorce, the birth of a sibling, or moving to a new home.

Stage Two: Borderline Stuttering (Ages 2–6)

The symptoms of borderline stuttering are:

- Disfluency on more than 10% of words.
- More than two disfluencies together ("That my-my-my ball").
- More repetitions and prolongations, and fewer revisions or incomplete phrases.
- No struggle behavior or fear of stuttering.

Stage Three: Beginning Stuttering (Ages 2–6)

At this stage, a child should be treated by a speech-language pathologist. The Stuttering Foundation of America has a videotape to help parents differentiate normal dysfluencies from beginning stuttering. The symptoms of beginning stuttering are:

- Part-word repetitions (not whole-word repetitions). Repetitions become rapid, tense, and irregular. A sound or word is repeated three or more times.
- The child substitutes the neutral or schwa vowel ("uh") instead of the appropriate vowel (e.g., "luh-luh-luh-like").
- Disfluency on more than 10% of words.
- The child stutters for weeks or months, between periods of fluency. Stuttering for more than six months is a danger sign.
- Stuttering when excited or upset, when having a great deal to say, or under high environmental demands.
- Prolongations. Sounds are prolonged at least a half-second. Fixed articulatory postures occur (freezing of speech-production muscles).
- Struggle and speech-production muscle tension, such as a rise in vocal pitch (caused by tensing the larynx), blocking airflow and stopping phonation, wide mouth opening or tongue protrusion, or irregular breathing patterns.
- Stuttering only on the first word of a sentence or phrase.
- Stuttering on both content and function words ("like," "but,"

"and," or "so").

- Secondary or escape behaviors, such as eye blinking, nodding, facial grimacing, quivering lip, raising eye brows, flaring nostrils.
- Frustration at being unable to get words out, but no fear or embarrassment about stuttering.

Stage Four: Intermediate Stuttering (Ages 6–13)

- Fear or avoidance of certain sounds or words. Word substitution begins.
- Blocks become common, in addition to repetitions and prolongations.
- Escape behaviors.
- Stuttering becomes chronic, without periods of fluency.
- Stuttering occurs on content words—major nouns, verbs, and adjectives.
- Stuttering varies among situations, such as talking on the telephone, speaking to strangers, or when excited.

Stage Five: Advanced Stuttering (Ages 14–Adult)

- Vivid, fearful anticipation of stuttering.
- Feared words, sounds, and situations.
- Thinks of himself as a stutterer. Chooses his friends, social activities, and jobs to avoid talking.
- Advanced stutterers may develop substitution and avoidance behaviors so well that you never know that they stutter.

Sudden Onset of Stuttering

The experts may be wrong that stuttering develops gradually in five stages. Some parents report that their children woke up one morning stuttering severely. These children went from normal dysfluencies to severe stuttering overnight. The children seem to have skipped the developmental stages in between.

And if stuttering has a genetic or neurological basis, then stuttering doesn't develop out of normal dysfluencies. (Instead, stuttering would develop from genetic or neurological abnormalities.) Brain scans have associated several neurological abnormalities with stuttering in adults, but no brain scans have been of stuttering children. Ideally, researchers would want brain scans of children before they stutter, and then brain scans after they begin stuttering. Perhaps some children are born with certain neurological abnormalities, which cause them to stutter when they learn to talk. If so, the "five stages" of stuttering development from normal dysfluencies is wrong. Or perhaps the "five stages" theory is right, and stuttering causes children's brains to grow abnormally. Or perhaps there's more than one type of stuttering in children, with more than one cause.

A Trigger for Tourette's

Tourette's syndrome is similar to stuttering in many ways. Persons with Tourette's syndrome have repetitive, semi-voluntary movements (tics) such as eye blinking, throat clearing, coughing, neck stretching, and shoulder shrugging. The tics are semi-voluntary in that tics can be consciously controlled, but this typically exacerbates the tics. Touretters often control the disorder by substituting more-acceptable tics. Different types of stress can set off or prevent bouts of tics. The same genes are associated with Tourette's and stuttering, and the same medications reduce both disorders. Tourette's has been described as "stuttering with one's hands and feet."

In a subgroup of individuals with Tourette's, a childhood auto-immune "trigger" led to Tourette's. A childhood streptococcal infection caused the child's immune system to attack brain cells in the putamen area.[91] The putamen controls gross (large) muscle movements. Excessive dopamine in the putamen area of the brain is associated with Tourette's. When the child recovered from the fever, he or she had Tourette's.

Could a child's immune system instead attack brain cells in the left caudate nucleus speech motor control area, and the child wakes up from an infection with severe stuttering? No researchers have investigated this question.

Direct and Indirect Therapy with Preschoolers

These questions aren't just "academic" musings. How children who stutter should be treated depends on the answers. The biggest issue in childhood stuttering treatment is direct vs. indirect therapy.

If children develop stuttering gradually from normal dysfluencies, then the ideal treatment would be early but mild. Speech-language pathologists would train parents to change their behavior, to reduce the stresses that cause dysfluent speech. Speech-language pathologists wouldn't directly change children's speech, because that would make the child believe that he or she was doing something wrong and so increase stress, which would increase stuttering. This is the position supporting *indirect therapy*.

On the other hand, if some children have a neurological predisposition to stuttering, a "gentle nudge" won't put them back onto the mainstream developmental track. These children will need a hard shove, or direct therapy.

Indirect Therapy

Indirect therapy is a "gentle nudge." Indirect therapy changes the *parents'* speech and behaviors. The speech-language pathologist trains the parents to slow down and use simple vocabulary, and not criticize the child, to not put pressure on the child (e.g., don't demand that the child confess guilt), to wait two seconds after the child finishes speaking before answering the child, and to give the child lots of hugs.

Indirect therapy is ineffective. A literature review found

> ...little convincing evidence...that parents of children who stutter differ from parents of children who do not stutter in the way they talk with their children. Similarly, there is little objective support...that parents' speech

behaviors contribute to children's stuttering or that modifying parents' speech behaviors facilitates children's fluency.[92]

More than a dozen studies found no evidence that altering parental behavior changed children's speech. These studies found no differences for:

- Positive statements (praise, encouragement, agreement).
- Negative statements (criticism, reprimands).
- Questions.
- Topic initiations and terminations.[93]
- Conversational assertiveness and responsiveness.[94]
- "Response time latency," or the time between one person finishing speaking and the other person beginning speaking.[95]
- "Formal" style vs. a "casual" style.[96]
- Illocution (the communicative effect of an utterance).[97]

Some studies found that indirect therapy produced results opposite to the researchers' intentions:

- A study found that mothers interrupt their child after dysfluencies, not before.[98] This suggests that *not* interrupting causes children to stutter!
- A study found that when mothers spoke faster their children spoke *slower*.[99] Another study trained parents to slow their speaking rates. The children's speaking rate *increased*.[100] This suggests that parents talking *slowly* causes their children to stutter!
- Parents of children who stutter produced more positive statements (e.g., praise, encouragement) and fewer negative statements (e.g. criticisms, disparaging remarks) than parents of children who didn't stutter.[101] This suggests that parents' praise and encouragement *causes* children to stutter!
- A multiyear study followed 93 preschool children. At the

start, none of the children stuttered. One year later, 26 of the children stuttered. The researchers compared the speech behaviors of the two groups of mothers, before their children started stuttering. No differences were found, except that mothers of children who would stutter had shorter, less complex utterances.[102] This contradicts the "capacities and demands model" of childhood stuttering.

More generally, some psychologists now discount the role of parents in the development of children's character and personality. About 50% of the personality differences are attributable to our genes, and the rest due to the child's peers: "...what parents do seems to be nearly irrelevant."[103]

Direct Therapy

In contrast, *direct therapy* changes the child's speech and behaviors. Direct therapy may include:

- Games to encourage speaking.
- Games to train specific speech skills, similar to adult fluency shaping therapy.
- Modeling the child's speech and/or behaviors.

A child's first therapy session may just be playing a game to encourage the child to talk. For example, the speech-language pathologist and child silently play with separate boxes of trucks, on opposite sides of the room. The speech-language pathologist begins making engine sounds. She then gradually moves to the center of the room, and her trucks interact with the child's trucks.

"Say the Magic Word" is another game to encourage talking. You can play this while looking through a picture book, or while driving. The parent says she sees something. The child guesses what the parent sees. When the child says the "magic word," the parent rings a bell or gives the child a peanut. No particular word is magic—the child is rewarded for fluent words.

A frequency-shifted auditory feedback (FAF) device (page 18) makes shy children want to talk. They're fascinated to hear their voices sounding like a "little kid" (frequency upshift) or a "monster" (frequency downshift).

Some games teach speech skills. In "Can't Catch Me," one person gets a peanut when the other person asks a question. You then quietly eat your peanut before answering the question. If you answer the question before eating your peanut, you must put your peanut back. The parent should lose more peanuts than the child, by answering too quickly. This reduces the time pressure the child feels about quickly answering questions.

A turtle hand puppet can teach slow speech with stretched vowels. When the child uses the target speech skills, the turtle slowly walks. When the child speaks fast, the turtle retreats into her shell.

The Super Duper catalog has other games for stuttering therapy (http://www.superduperinc.com/).

Modeling

> Caitlyn, a four-year-old female who began to stutter in the midst of her parents' divorce, was exhibiting significant struggle and tension behavior as well as secondary behaviors. Of most concern was her head-banging behavior during difficult moments of stuttering. After many sessions in which I attempted to eliminate this behavior through fluency-shaping principles, I saw no change. One day, shortly after Caitlyn banged her forehead on the table to interrupt a block, I modeled the same behavior. Caitlyn was shocked and ignored me. After I did this several times she asked me, "Why did you do that? Didn't that hurt?" I responded, "I don't know why I did it. But it sure didn't help me get my word out!" Caitlyn never again banged her head to help her talk. She has been out of therapy for six years and remains fluent.[104]

This speech-language pathologist's *modeling* of Caitlyn's behavior was radically different from conventional stuttering therapy practices. The speech-language pathologist improved the child's awareness of her stuttering. In contrast, most "experts" would have pretended not to notice Caitlyn's head-banging behavior. They would have predicted that making Caitlyn aware of her head-banging would have caused emotional trauma and made her stuttering worse.

Imagine that a teenage brother and sister use profanity at the family dinner table. Should the parents act horrified and tell their children never to use such language? Should they refuse to allow dessert or television for the teenagers?

You know that won't work. The teenagers will use profanity at the next opportunity, just for the amusement of horrifying their parents. Instead, the parents should immediately use twice as much profanity. Dad should say, "#$%^, this is best *&^% meatloaf in the whole @#$% world!"

Mom should then respond, "Oh, you big !@#$, you're so #$%^ sexy and when you talk ^%$#!"

I guaranty that the teenagers will turn red with embarrassment, and never use profanity again in front of their parents.

In a psychology class about traumatized children we saw a video of a ten-year-old boy destroying a psychologist's office. The boy threw every object he could throw, and smashed everything else. The psychologist sat there calmly telling the boy not to destroy the office. He finally grabbed the boy and hugged him. To me it looked like a full body restraint but the instructor said it was a hug, and that was what the boy really needed. I asked what would have happened if the psychologist had modeled the boy's behavior. For example, the psychologist could have thrown and smashed stuff. The instructor said that was the worst idea she'd ever heard. But I think the boy would have stopped, watched in amazement as the psychologist destroyed his own office, and then asked, "Why did you do that?" The boy and the psychologist could then have started talking, with understanding of what the boy was feeling, which is what I think the boy needed.

The purpose of modeling is to improve the subject's awareness of his or her behaviors. Stutterers are largely unaware of their stuttering, or at least what they do when they stutter. Everyone else can see the stuttering but the stutterer can't. Combining video and modeling can help a stutterer improve self-awareness.

Modeling also dispels a person's mistaken view that a behavior is invisible, or it's acceptable, or everyone does it. If everyone ignores undesirable behavior then the person may think it's OK.

Modeling only works when the modeler or the modelee knows how to replace the undesirable behavior with a target behavior. For example, it's OK for your speech-language pathologist to model your stuttering because she can show you how to speak fluently. It was OK for my Romantic Disaster of 1996 (page 64) to make me aware that I was stuttering, because I knew what to do to talk fluently. It's not OK to point out a problem to someone who has no idea what to do about it.

School-Age Stuttering

Ask your child whether he or she likes school. When I was in elementary school, the girls liked school and the boys didn't. At this age, girls see school as where they socialize with their friends, via quiet verbal communication and cooperation.

Boys see school as where they're told *not* to play with their friends, via physical interaction such as running around or showing off their physical abilities. This difference makes school more stressful for boys, with effects on their speech.

Why Do More Boys Than Girls Stutter?

Among preschoolers, boys who stutter outnumber girls who stutter about two to one, or fewer.[105]

But more girls recover fluent speech, and more boys don't.[106] By fifth grade the ratio is about four boys who stutter to one girl who stutters. This ratio remains into adulthood.[107]

Why boys are more likely to stutter, and less likely to recover, isn't certain. Boys generally have more diseases and disorders, for reasons having to do with the Y chromosome (the Y chromosome has fewer genes than the X chromosome so the two chromosomes pair incompletely). Boys generally have more speech disorders because girls are usually better at speech and language, and especially at using speech and language for social purposes. Speech and language tend to be more stressful for boys, so boys usually prefer to interact physically.

I suspect that girls' develop the ability to socialize with other children in groups by age five, but boys develop this ability later. This was apparent to me at my nephew's sixth birthday party. One of his presents was a slinky. I showed his friends how to make the slinky walk down stairs. Three girls sat together at the top of the stairs and took turns. One girl could easily make the slinky walk down the stairs. This was harder for the second girl, but she could do it. The third girl couldn't do it at all. But they cooperated and encouraged each other.

Two boys wanted to try it. But they couldn't get to top of the stairs without wrestling each other and falling back down the stairs. I wouldn't allow wrestling on the stairs, so they'd run around the living room chasing each other. Then they'd come back to play with the slinky, but start wrestling on the stairs again.

At five, girls are ready to start school. Boys are wild animals until seven. School can be stressful for boys who aren't ready for school. The most stressful part of school for boys may be the communication demands. Girls are using communication to make friends. Girls' communication skills and social skills develop together. In contrast, boys may not be ready to socialize with 25 other children, in a building with hundreds of other children. Some children are in school and day care for twelve hours, without time to relax or to be alone—that'd stress me out!

If your five- or six-year-old son stutters, and you don't think he's ready for school (e.g., he vomits or wets his pants at school), consider keeping him home another year, or look into a co-op school where a parent can attend school with him, or let him attend school but don't put him in daycare for another six hours each day.

Motivation for Speech Therapy
The father of a ten-year-old stutterer wanted to do everything to

help his son. On the advice of his son's speech-language pathologist, the father bought my company's top-of-the-line electronic stuttering therapy device. The speech-language pathologist trained the father to use the device. The father worked with his son thirty minutes every evening.

After two months, the father returned the device for a refund. The son was 100% fluent when practicing with the device. The kid had no interest in using slow, relaxed speech the rest of the day. Stuttering didn't stop the boy from playing baseball or doing other things boys do. In the world of seven- to twelve-year-old boys, talking isn't an important activity.

But your seven- to twelve-year-old son's good self-esteem can be a double-edged sword. It's hard to get school-age boys motivated to do speech therapy. This makes it more important that parents do speech therapy with their child in every conversation. Ask your child's speech-language pathologist what your child should be doing (e.g., slow speech with stretched vowels). Have your child use therapy skills on every sentence he says to you. Be your child's therapy helper.

SLPs vs. Parents vs. Computers

A study of 98 children, 9 to 14 years old, compared three types of stuttering therapy.[108] The three types of therapy were:

- Intensive "smooth speech" fluency shaping trained relaxed, diaphragmatic breathing; a slow speaking rate with prolonged vowels; gentle onsets and offsets (loudness contour); soft articulation contacts; and pauses between phrases. The children did this therapy in a speech clinic for 35 hours over one week.

- Home-based "smooth speech." This was similar to the first group, but parents were included, and encouraged to continue therapy at home. Therapy was done in a speech clinic for six hours once a week for four weeks (24 hours total).

- Electromyographic biofeedback. The children used an EMG

biofeedback computer system about six hours a day for one week (30 hours total). The EMG system monitored the child's speech-production muscle activity. The children were instructed to tense and then relax their speech-production muscles. The goal was to develop awareness and control of these muscles. The children then worked through a hierarchy from simple words to conversations, while keeping their speech-production muscles relaxed. After mastering this while watching the computer display, the children did the exercises with the computer monitoring but not displaying their muscle activity. The speech pathologists did relatively little with the children: "Constant clinician presence was not necessary as the computer provided feedback as to whether the child was performing the skills correctly."

- A fourth (control) group didn't receive any stuttering therapy.

At the end of each therapy program, all three therapies reduced stuttering below 1% on average. The control group had no improvement in fluency.

One year after the therapy program, the percentage of children with disfluency rates under 2% were:

- 48% of the children from the clinician-based program.
- 63% of the children from the parent-based program.
- 71% of the children from the computer-based program.

The results for children with disfluency rates under 1% were even more striking:

- 10% of the children from the clinician-based program.
- 37% of the children from the "parent-based" program.
- 44% of the children from the computer-based program.

In other words, the computers were most effective, the parents next most effective, and the speech-language pathologists were least effective in the long term. At the 1% disfluency level, the computers and the parents were about four times more effective than the speech-language pathologists.

Four years later, all three groups had average stuttering reductions between 76% and 79%. This may have been due to the more dysfluent children receiving additional speech therapy.[109]

Advice for Parents, by Magdalene Lima, SLP

A survey of school speech-language pathologists found that that less than 25% of the children treated were considered to be recovered. The children were treated for an average of three years.[110] These aren't stellar results.

A school speech-language pathologist about her experiences:

I am a speech-language pathologist in private practice and formerly a public school therapist for nine years. My suggestions to parents of children with speech problems are:

Do some research in these areas. Check out the communication disorders websites.

Go to your school speech-language pathologist with what you know and ask her what she thinks. The best approach is to treat her as the professional she is in a non-critical way with the attitude that you just want to understand all the treatments available for your son. Offer to help get information to her if she doesn't have it. Let her know you understand the position she is in and that you are on her team. This will get you much further in getting the appropriate services for your child than fighting your school.

If your insurance covers it or you have the funds, find a good private pediatric speech and language clinic in your area and AT LEAST have an evaluation done. Just that information alone could really help the school SLP. If you can afford private therapy, get it. The main difference in service is that your child will receive individual therapy with a clinician that has the time and resources needed to provide the highest quality therapy.

As a former school speech-language pathologist, my skills and knowledge didn't suddenly change when I switched over to private practice. The setting changed, and that makes a huge difference. I now serve 30 clients rather than 75, I see them all individually, and I am paid more than in the schools. In the hours I don't see clients, I am busy researching, giving parent support, writing regular and detailed reports, and planning innovative therapy rather than going to bus duty, lunch duty, hall duty, faculty meetings that don't really apply to me and filling out massive amounts of government-required paperwork.

Is The Problem Ability or Setting?

Now to those of you who think the worst of the public school speech-language pathologist: I'd like you to stand in her shoes for a minute. In the last three years of my public school experience my caseload became unmanageable. I had 75 students, including a severely and profoundly handicapped class, four autistic students and all other students in speech from grades K-5 at that school. I begged, cried and pleaded for help from my supervisors. I KNEW I could not provide the quality of service each and every one of these students and their families deserved. However, the answer was always: get creative, we don't have money in the budget. Please understand, in my situation, it was not a lack of caring, lack of skill or ability—there was absolutely nothing I could do. I became angry and frustrated at our administration. Why didn't they provide the training, time, personnel and support we needed to provide services to these students?

Speech Pathology: A Growing and Diverse Field

The disorders in our field and the therapies that have now been developed have become extremely specialized. In the schools I was expected by parents to be an expert in the following fields: stuttering, swallowing disorders, voice disorders, articulation disorders including tongue thrust, cleft palate, phonological process disorders as well as motor speech disorders, autism and PDD, traumatic brain injury, ADHD, language and learning disabilities, hearing impairments and social and pragmatic communication disorders. Excuse me, do you realize that just as physicians receive a basic foundation in medicine, so do speech-language pathologists receive a basic foundation in all of the above disorders. You graduate from college and through your experience and personal growth and research, you become an expert in a few areas. It would be virtually impossible for one person to have the time and energy it would take to become an expert in all those areas!

This is why our field is moving towards specialty certifications. What will public schools do then? I guess they will have to hire the specialists that their individual students require.

Many and Varied Problems in the Schools
More and more our district began hiring speech assistants (speech practitioners who are not required to meet the standards of education, clinical practicum and experience needed to be fully certified and licensed) to handle huge caseloads with minimal supervision from licensed speech-language pathologists. There is a shortage of qualified speech language pathologists willing to go into public school therapy when there are much more lucrative and attractive positions available in other settings. As I talked with administrators, I soon became aware of the pressure being applied to them from the state, parents and other agencies to meet all these educational requirements. For every parent who complains there is not enough money to provide quality special education services in the school, there is another parent complaining that their gifted and talented child is not being given the education THEY deserve because of all the money being poured into special education programs. Or what about the parents of children in sports programs, they have THEIR list of complaints. Everyone thinks that their cause is totally justified because they are arguing for their children, and nothing can convince anyone that their child doesn't deserve the best.

I left the public school system to go into private practice and now my problem is solved—I love my work and I'm giving quality services to clients with fantastic results! However, what's your solution? My final and personal resolution to this whole issue, is that in many cases—not all, but many—I truly feel that schools are doing the very best they can with the resources available to them to provide the services that our children need. However, sometimes, parents are right, it's not enough. So what are we going to do? Is every parent in America with a complaint going to file suit against the local school district? If this happens, our schools will begin focusing on preventing lawsuits rather than on how best to serve and educate our children.

Work With Your Administration/Educators
Sometimes all it takes is going to an administrator, such as the Director of Special Education, and pleading your case. Also give your specific suggestions at your child's IEP meeting. You'd better have some research and documentation to back up the necessity of your suggestions. The attitude and manner in which you present yourself is of utmost importance, if they perceive you are willing to make compromises and work with them they will be more willing to stick their neck out for you. Suggest specific things such as the district paying for an outside assessment, or hiring a consultant temporarily who can lend their expertise to your child's case. Get over any intimidation you feel in asserting yourself with these people, they are just people with children and jobs and stresses just like you. What they say to you is never written in stone.

Conclusion
I'm not saying you shouldn't fight extreme injustice or abuse. I'm saying it's a huge system with a lot of variables involved. The fight is societal and governmental—usually not your local educational facility. Become involved politically in your state with your speech and hearing association—they always have a branch that is lobbying for legislation to improve speech services in the schools. Meanwhile, you have a child that has needs for quality services in the area of speech pathology, do the best you can to get that service, whether it be private therapy through insurance or private

pay, or school therapy, don't stop looking until you find what you need.

YOU take responsibility to research, learn things for yourself and communicate with those who affect your child's education.

Fostering Teenagers' Passion for Fluency

I am a mother of a stuttering thirteen-year-old boy. Stuttering really had never bothered him until this year. It is very frustrating for him to talk on the phone. His friends call all the time but he has refrained from talking on the phone because his stuttering seems to get worse. My husband and I have noticed him withdrawing from his peers. We have always had an active role with his stuttering. He has been to a lot of speech-language pathologists and we have also tried the CAFET [biofeedback computer] system. This was helping him. Unfortunately the closest center was more than two hours away. After one year it was too stressful on him missing too much school. Because of this we had to stop. Since then he has wanted nothing to do with speech-language pathologists.

I hear similar stories about other teenagers, with these elements:
- The teenager has been seeing his school's speech-language pathologists for five or even ten years. His speech isn't improving. He wants to discontinue speech therapy.
- He's fluent in the speech-language pathologist's office, but stutters everywhere else.
- The parents have taken him to other speech clinics, without success.
- He used to have good speech attitudes, saying whatever he wanted. Now he fears and avoids certain words or speaking situations.
- His social behavior has changed. He's withdrawing from social contacts.

Previously he saw himself as being like most other kids, doing the same things as other kids. School-age boys' social activities, e.g., baseball, don't demand much talking. Now he thinks of himself as a stutterer, different from other teenagers. Teenagers' social activities, e.g., dating or getting an after-school job, are harder for a stutterer.

Your teenager is an adult, in terms of stuttering. He should be doing adult stuttering therapy. This can include:

- Psychological stuttering therapy, training fluent speech (physical) skills.
- A support group for teenagers who stutter.
- An intensive speech therapy program or a summer camp for teenagers who stutter. (Google "speech camp for teens who stutter.")

Develop a Passion

In the chapter "Famous People Who Stutter" (page 139), you'll learn that many actors and singers developed their talents during high school as a result of stuttering. When a teenager feels passion for an activity, he or she can focus with greater intensity than adults. Your job, as a parent, is to help your teenager focus on a speech-positive activity, instead of focusing on video games or memorizing Black Sabbath lyrics.

Help your teenager become passionately involved in activities that require talking, improve his fluency, and develop his social skills. Such activities include:

- Singing.
- Acting.
- Debating.
- Foreign languages.
- Organizing a teenage stuttering support group.

Or do a science project about stuttering. See

http://en.wikibooks.org/wiki/Speech-Language_Pathology/Stuttering/High_School_Science_Projects

Involve Peers in Speech Therapy

Are your teenage clients less than enthusiastic about speech therapy? Well, duh, if you're a speech-language pathologist then you're at least 25! You might even be over 30! Why would a teenage want to talk to someone so old?

Instead, have a teenager bring a friend to speech therapy. He'll talk to his friend about skateboarding or video games or other stuff you're clueless about. Better yet, you can train the friend to give your client a subtle reminder when he needs to slow down or get back on-target (see "My Romantic Disaster of 1996," page 64).

Or roleplay teenage situations, such as different ways of asking a peer out on a date.

Paramount in teenagers' minds is connecting to peers (other teenagers), e.g., being seen as "cool" by their classmates. Use speech therapy as a way to connect to peers and your teenager will want to do speech therapy. For example, instead of (thinking of himself as) being seen as a boy who stutters, help your teenager think of himself as a boy who's not afraid to ask girls for their telephone numbers and ask them out on dates.

Learn American Sign Language

I took four years of German in high school and college. The classes were taught in a conversational style. Being unable to talk, I learned nothing.

No one suggested that I study American Sign Language instead. I could have been 100% fluent in that! Being good at something would have improved my self-esteem. In contrast, I felt like the stupidest person in the German classes. And if I learned sign language I would've made friends in the deaf community, or maybe worked part-time as a sign language interpreter.

Famous People Who Stutter

Stuttering is a difficult and demoralizing disability, but with persistence many stutterers overcome the disorder and go on to successful lives.

Singers and Actors

Some stutterers are afraid to open their mouths. But other stutterers earn their living with their voices.

Carly Simon, Singer-Songwriter

Carly Simon (1945-) began stuttering severely when she was eight years old. She blames her stuttering on her then 44-year-old mother's affair with their 20-year-old live-in tennis instructor. The affair caused jealousy, anger, "lies and a train of deception" in the Simons' affluent household.

A psychiatrist tried unsuccessfully to cure Simon's stuttering. Instead, Simon turned to singing and songwriting. "I felt so strangulated talking that I did the natural thing, which is to write songs, because I could sing without stammering, as all stammerers can."[111]

Simon wrote some of the most-loved songs of the 1970s, including "Anticipation" and "You're So Vain." She won an Oscar and a Grammy. She was married to James Taylor for nine years. They have two children.

Mel Tillis, Country Music Entertainer

As a child, Mel Tillis (1932-), was laughed at because he stuttered.[112] He said to himself, "Well, if they're gonna laugh at me, then I'll give them something to laugh about."

In 1957 he began working as a singer for Minnie Pearl, Nashville's great country comedienne. Pearl encouraged Tillis to talk on stage, but he refused, afraid that he'd be laughed at.

Pearl replied, "Let 'em laugh. Goodness gracious, laughs are hard to get and I'm sure that they're laughing with you and not against you, Melvin."

Little by little, Tillis increased his speaking on-stage. He developed humorous routines about his stuttering. Then "word began to circulate around Nashville about this young singer from Florida who could write songs and sing, but stuttered like hell when he tried to talk. The next thing I knew I was being asked to be on every major television show in America." Tillis' career took off.

But before Nashville and fame and fortune, Tillis was looking for a job in Florida. No one hired him. At the last place he applied, the owner said that he had once stuttered. He wouldn't hire Tillis, but gave him a piece of paper to read every night, saying that it had changed his life.

On the paper was a prayer:

> Oh Lord, Grant me the Courage to change the things I can change, the Serenity to accept those I cannot change, and the Wisdom to know the difference. And God, Grant me the Courage to not give up on what I think is right, even though I think it is hopeless.

Tillis concludes his story,

> For the first time in a long time, I slept well that night. I woke the next morning with a different outlook on life. I told myself that if I couldn't quit stuttering, then the world was going to have to take me like I was. What you see is what you get. From that day on, things started looking up for Mel Tillis. Soon after, I headed for Nashville in a '49 Mercury with a wife and a four-month-old baby girl—her name was Pam.

Tillis was 1976 Country Music Entertainer of the Year.

James Earl Jones, Actor

James Earl Jones (1931-), the most in-demand voice in Holly-wood, is a stutterer.

Jones was "virtually mute" as a child.[113] With the help of his high school English teacher, Jones overcame stuttering by reading Shakespeare "aloud in the fields to myself," and then reading to audiences, and then acting.

Jones is proudest of his role as Shakespeare's *Othello*, but is best-known as the voice of Darth Vader in *Star Wars*. He recently portrayed a stutterer in the movie *A Family Thing* (1995).

Peter Bonerz, Director

Peter Bonerz (1938-), who played Jerry the dentist on *The Bob Newhart Show*, and directed *Friends*, *Murphy Brown*, and *Home Improvement*, said about his stuttering:[114]

> I'm 58 years old, and if I stutter while giving Candice Bergen a direction, who cares? If (the stuttering) is really difficult, I exaggerate it and get everyone on the set to laugh with me. A stutter can really be quite charming. We are human and not perfect.

Athletes

Some stutterers compensate for their speech difficulties by excel-ling at non-verbal activities, such as sports. But you'll see that top athletes must do more than score points in a game.

Bob Love, Basketball Player

Bob Love (1942-) was a three-time NBA All-Star and led the Chicago Bulls in scoring for seven consecutive seasons. Reporters rarely interviewed him. "I would score 45 points, go into the locker room, and all the reporters would come down," Love recalls. "Everybody would pass me by."

Love retired in 1977. Because of his stuttering he went from one dead-end job to another. The low point was in 1985, at the age of 42, when a restaurant hired Love as a $4.45/hour busboy. Love had tried speech therapy twice before without success. He tried again. After a year of stuttering therapy, Love began public speaking. As a boy, he had a dream of standing on a podium, speaking to thousands of people. Love gave motivational speeches to churches, high school students, and other groups. He's now director of community relations and spokesman for the Bulls. "It's hard to believe I make a living speaking. It's a dream come true. I held onto my dreams, and I tell kids they have to hold on to theirs."[115]

Bill Walton, Basketball Player
Bill Walton (1952-) led UCLA to two NCAA titles, and the Portland Trailblazers and Boston Celtics to NBA championships. His stuttering was so severe that he couldn't say simple phrases like "thank you."

Today, Walton has overcome his stuttering and works as a sports commentator for NBC Sports.

As Walton was battling stuttering through childhood, college, and his professional career, he used basketball as a sanctuary, a place where he didn't have to think about his speech. The challenges in his personal life pushed him to become one of the best players on the court.

Amazingly, on the court, he could not only play ball, he could speak, too. Or at least yell. "I never had any trouble yelling at the refs," Walton said. "In the heat of the game…when it was just totally spontaneous, I could get out there and really scream and yell at the refs. But it was only in basketball, and it was only at the refs."

When each game ended, Walton stuttered again.

"During college, the teasing was tough," he said. "I had a speech class one year, and they laughed me out of the class." It didn't matter to his classmates that he was the college basketball Player of the Year. "I was trying to make it in school, and they just laughed me out of the class."

At awards ceremonies and media events, Walton shied away

from microphones. He even had other people speak on his behalf. "When I had to actually formulate words and make a statement, I could not do it at all," he recalls.

In the NBA, he faced some of the toughest and most legendary players in the history of the game. Playing basketball with Kareem Abdul-Jabbar and Larry Bird came naturally. Speaking, still, did not.

After he retired from basketball, the sanctuary was gone. The hiding place that had protected him for 28 years could shelter him no longer. But his love for the game helped him with stuttering.

According to Walton, long-time friend and Hall of Fame broadcaster Marty Glickman pulled him aside at a social event and said, "You've got to learn how to talk."

"He gave me some very basic tips, and I applied those tips to the learning techniques I learned from my coach at UCLA John Wooden about how to develop as a basketball player," Walton explained. "I thought about fundamentals and how to start with the basics like the ability to mechanically duplicate moves on the basketball court. And I just applied that to speaking."

So Walton learned to speak, just as he had learned basketball years before. Not only did he stop stuttering, he found a way back —through sports commentating—to the game he loved so much.

When he began broadcasting for NBC Sports, all of his fears resurfaced. Off the court, he was still afraid to talk. He describes his first broadcast as "painful" but knows now that the worst is over. "I used to be really embarrassed about stuttering. But now I realize that it's something that is a part of me...something that I have to deal with and work on every day. If I don't work on it, I'm not going to be able to do my job. It's always a challenge," Walton said. He doesn't mind the challenge—that's what makes him strive to do his best.

Walton challenges others to get on top of stuttering too. "It's important to know that help is out there. The ability to learn how to talk is easily the greatest thing I've ever done. Winning two NCAA championships and two NBA titles was nice, but I knew it was going to happen. But learning how to speak has given me a whole new life. I have been set free."[116]

Bo Jackson

Baseball and football pro Bo Jackson (1962-) wrote:

> My teachers thought I couldn't read. I could read, but I'd never read aloud because I stuttered. The other kids would laugh at me, and I became a recluse. I was angry at myself and at them, and it often resulted in my beating someone up after school. I had to live with it for eight or nine years, but I finally decided to pay it no attention and forced myself to do everything from reading in class to making speeches. Eventually, I learned to relax and take my time.[117]

Writers and Photographers

Essayist Thomas Carlyle wrote of novelist and stutterer Henry James (1843-1916), author of *Portrait of a Lady* and *Turn of the Screw*: "A stammering man is never a worthless one...It is an excess of delicacy, excess of sensibility to the presence of his fellow-creature, that makes him stammer."[118]

Contemporary fiction authors who stutter include horror writer Peter Straub[119] (1943- ; *Shadowland, Ghost Story*); mystery writer Paul Johnson (*Killing The Blues*),[120] and David Shields (*Dead Languages* includes a funny short story about his childhood experiences in school speech therapy). John Updike (1932- ; the *Rabbit* series, *Brazil*) believes that his stuttering is precipitated when "I feel myself in a false position," such as guilt of being "in the wrong."[121]

Nature writer and editor Edward Hoagland (*The Snow Leopard*) not only stutters, but was blind for several years. He wrote of this experience in *Tigers & Ice*. Zoologist Alan Rabinowitz's book *Beyond The Last Village* (2002) recounts his explorations in Asia searching for endangered wildlife, and his experiences stuttering.[122]

Benson Bobrick has written popular histories of the English

Bible, the American Revolution, Russia and Siberia, and a history of stuttering, *Knotted Tongues* (1995).

Marty Jezer (died 2005) wrote a history of the 1950s, biographies of Abbie Hoffman and Rachel Carson, and an autobiography, *Stuttering: A Life Bound Up In Words* (1997).

Publishers who stutter include Henry Luce (1898-1967), founder of *Time* magazine and *Sports Illustrated*; and Walter Annenberg (1908-2002), founder of *TV Guide* and *Seventeen*. In 1993, Annenberg donated $500 million to improve American schools.[123]

Photographers

Howard Bingham, friend of Muhammed Ali and O.J. Simpson, stuttered as a witness in Simpson's trial. Growing up, Bingham "endured the usual teasing from schoolmates because of his stuttering. In high school…he hid behind his stuttering and didn't volunteer for anything."

Bingham's friendship with Muhammed Ali began in 1962, continued through photographing the Black Panther Party and "virtually every significant urban uprising" in the 1960s. Bingham later worked as Bill Cosby's photographer. He wrote the book *Muhammed Ali: A Thirty Year Journey*, and worked for years to get his friend the honor of lighting the Olympic flame that started the 1996 Atlanta Games. Ironically, Bingham now sometimes has to talk for Ali, due to Ali having Parkinson's disease.[124]

Political and Business Leaders

Annie Glenn (1920-), wife of astronaut and Senator John Glenn, once refused to talk to President Johnson because of her stuttering.[125]

Representative Dennis Kucinich (1946- ; D-Ohio) overcame stuttering as a child. Rep. Kucinich was elected mayor of Cleveland at the age of 31. As a state senator, he won the 1996 National Association for Social Workers Outstanding Senator of the Year

Award. He also won an Emmy for his political analysis television broadcasts.[126]

Other political leaders who stutter include Berkeley Free Speech leader Mario Savio[127] (1942-1996) and congressman Frank Wolf (1939- ; R-Virginia).[128]

Business Leaders

In the business world, John Sculley's (1939-) stuttering "has taken him many years to overcome. He was also painfully shy."

Sculley wrote in his autobiography, "I was determined to build a strength out of what was originally a weakness. I went to the theater to watch how performers positioned themselves on stage. I'd practice for hours. I became obsessed with the idea that I was going to become better than anyone else as a business communicator."[129]

Sculley rose to president of Pepsi-Cola. He succeeded in overtaking Coca-Cola as the #1 soft drink. He then changed coasts and cultures to become president of Apple Computer for ten years. Sculley became a great public speaker, gaining "renown for his ability to deliver rousing speeches in front of thousands, sometimes without notes."[130]

Sidney Gottlieb, CIA Spook

The man who brought us LSD was "a lifelong stutterer." Sidney Gottlieb (1918-1999), described by friends as "a kind of genius," had a Ph.D. in biochemistry from Caltech. He joined the CIA in 1951. In 1953 he founded the MKUltra program, which gave LSD to thousands of CIA agents, military officers, college students, prisoners, and mental patients. Many of the study participants were unknowingly dosed with the drug. Gottlieb took LSD hundreds of times.

Gottlieb's later work at the CIA included developing "a poison handkerchief to kill an Iraqi colonel, an array of toxic gifts to be delivered to Fidel Castro, and a poison dart to kill a leftist leader in the Congo. None of the plans succeeded."

After leaving the CIA, Gottlieb became a speech-language pathologist, then raised goats on a commune in Virginia.[131]

British Royalty and Commoners

Several British royals stuttered. Charles I (1600-1649) was king from 1625 until 1649, during the English Civil War. His inability to speak to Parliament "had an unfavorable influence on his affairs." Charles lost the war and was executed. It didn't help that he proclaimed that he was above the law: "a king and a subject are two plain different things." His father, James I (1566-1625), was described as "having a tongue too big for his mouth"—possibly an articulation disorder.[132]

George VI (1895-1952) was king from 1937 until 1952. He was father of Queen Elizabeth II. His annual live Christmas broadcasts were "always an ordeal."[133] Robert Graves' 1937 novel *I, Claudius* is ostensibly about the Roman emperor Claudius, who stuttered. But the personality and life of Graves' Claudius were taken from the shy George VI. George survived the scandals of his brother Edward's abdication, was thrust into a role to which he was thought unsuited, and surprised everyone by becoming one of the most capable and loved modern kings.

Winston Churchill and Aneurin Bevan, Statesmen

Sixty years ago the best orators of the British Parliament were both stutterers. Aneurin Bevan (1897-1960), leader of the Labour Party and architect of the National Health Service, forced himself to make speeches as often as possible. He spoke fluently when his passions were aroused, so he spoke passionately for British workers in the 1930s. Bevan developed an extraordinary vocabulary by substituting words to avoid stuttering.[134]

Winston Churchill (1874-1965), leader of the Conservative Party, could speak fluently only by preparing his remarks in advance. He studied issues weeks in advance, and wrote out responses to any possible objection. This extra effort made Churchill more knowledgeable than other leaders.[135]

As a young man, Churchill worried that his stuttering would have an impact upon his ambition to go into politics. But he didn't believe in submitting to failure so he practiced and persevered. He both practiced his speeches and practiced nonsense phrases as he walked, such as "The Spanish ships I cannot see since they are not in sight." When he was 23, he wrote, "Sometimes a slight and not unpleasing stammer or impediment has been of some assistance in securing the attention of the audience..."[136]

More British Stutterers

The British are fond of eccentrics and stutterers.[137]

Erasmus Darwin (1731-1802) was a physician and naturalist and was invited to be the personal physician for King George III of England.[138] His grandson, naturalist Charles Darwin (1809-1882), also stuttered.

Charles Canon Kingsley (1819-1875) was a Cambridge history professor, orator, and chaplain to Queen Victoria. His novels include the popular pirate adventure *Westward, Ho!* and the popular children's book *The Water-Babies*. He recommended treating stuttering with a "manly" diet of beef and beer.

Charles Lutwidge Dodgson (1832-1898) was an Oxford mathematician, minister, and photographer. On July 4, 1862, while boating on the Thames, he told a friend's children, including a daughter named Alice, a story of a girl named Alice. Dodgson later published *Alice's Adventures in Wonderland* under the pen name Lewis Carroll.

Somerset Maugham (1874-1965) was the highest-paid writer of the 1930s. His novels include *The Razor's Edge* and *The Moon and Sixpence*. In his autobiographical novel *Of Human Bondage* he substituted a clubfoot for his stuttering, because stuttering was too difficult to transcribe in writing.

Lord David Cecil (1902-1986) was Professor of English literature at Oxford in the 1950s. "Lord David's stutter was thought of as a mark of high-bred diffidence...As an Oxford undergraduate in the fifties, I expected my tutors to stutter; it was their way of not *insisting*, I thought, and very Oxford." John Bailey, husband of novelist Iris Murdoch and another student of Lord David Cecil, also stutters.[139]

Kim Philby (1912-1988) was a spy. Stuttering once saved his life, by confounding a fast-paced interrogator.

Patrick Campbell (1913-1980) was a British humorist and 3rd Baron Glenavy. He wrote, "From my earliest days I have enjoyed an attractive impediment in my speech. I have never permitted the use of the word 'stammer.' I can't say it myself."[140]

Margaret Drabble (1939-) is the editor of *The Oxford Companion to English Literature*. Her novels include *The Seven Sisters* and *The Red Queen*.

In the Ancient World

Stuttering is one of the few disorders that generally gets better over time. Most children who stutter outgrow it. Even adults who stutter severely in their teens and 20s often overcome stuttering—via speech therapy or on their own—in their 30s or 40s. At the life stage when other people experience the dreams of their youth crashing down, stutterers realize they can accomplish anything they want, regardless of their speech. Stutterers are less likely to be famous in their youth, and more likely to be famous five hundred years later.

Moses, Israelite Leader
Or five thousand years later. Moses stuttered:

> But Moses said to the Lord, "Oh, my Lord, I am not eloquent, either heretofore or since thou hast spoken to thy servant; but I am slow of speech and of tongue."
> Then the Lord said to him, "Who has made man's mouth? Who makes him dumb, or deaf, or seeing, or blind? Or who gives sight to one and makes another blind? Is it not I, the Lord? Now, therefore go, and I will

be with your mouth and teach you what you shall speak."

But he said, "Oh, my Lord, send, I pray, some other person."

Then the anger of the Lord was kindled against Moses and he said, "Is there not Aaron, your brother, the Levite? I know that he can speak well; and behold, he is coming out to meet you, when he sees you he will be glad in his heart. And you shall speak to him and put the words in his mouth; and I will be with your mouth and with his mouth, and will teach you what you shall do. He shall speak for you to the people; and he shall be a mouth for you, and he shall be to him as God."[141]

Aesop, Master Storyteller

Aesop (620 to 560 BC) was born a slave and "most deformed" and "he coulde not speke." One day he fell asleep under a shady tree. The Goddess of Hospitality appeared to him in a dream and gave him the gift of speech. His life changed and he became a master storyteller.[142]

Demosthenes, Orator

Demosthenes (384 BC–322 BC) was the greatest orator of ancient Greece. He overcame stuttering by speaking with pebbles in his mouth to improve articulation, shouting above the ocean waves to improve his volume, and working with an actor in reciting Sophocles and Euripedes to coordinate his voice and gestures.[143]

Virgil, Poet

Publius Vergilius Maro (70 BC-19 BC), known in English as Virgil or Vergil, was a Roman poet. His works included the *Eclogues*, the *Georgics* and the *Aeneid*, the latter becoming the Roman Empire's national epic poem.

Claudius, Emperor

Tiberius Claudius Caesar Augustus Germanicus (10 BC-AD 54), was the Roman Emperor from AD 41 to AD 54.

Claudius stuttered severely and was said to have weak hands

and knees, although he was a tall, well-built man with no physical disability. His symptoms diminished after he became emperor. Claudius said that he'd exaggerated his weaknesses to avoid being murdered. By appearing to be weak and disabled, Claudius survived the deaths of rivals to the throne. He then served as one of the most effective and able emperors of Rome, for thirteen years.

Claudius' life was portrayed in Robert Graves' novel *I, Claudius* (1934), which was made into a television series in 1976.

Dekanawida, The Great Peacemaker

Dekanawida invented representative federal government. He united the Iroquois nations in what is now New York State, in the sixteenth century, before the Iroquois encountered Europeans.

The Iroquois federation was a model, thanks to Ben Franklin's experience making treaties with the Iroquois, for the Americans and French to create representative federal democracies.

> The League of the Five Nations of the Iroquois was established, according to eighteenth-century sources, in the late sixteenth century. Iroquois tradition tells of constant warfare...One bereaved by this warfare was a Mohawk man, Hiawatha ("He Who Makes Rivers").
>
> Crazed by grief for his murdered family, Hiawatha fled into the forests, living like a cannibal monster in the Iroquois myths. One day, Hiawatha met Dekanawida. The charismatic goodness of this man, said to have been a Huron miraculously born of a virgin, reawakened in Hiawatha his humanity.
>
> Dekanawida confided to Hiawatha plans to free their peoples from the horrors of war by allying all the Iroquois in a grand league, a longhouse...in which [the leader of] each Iroquois nation would sit as a brother with brothers.
>
> The visionary felt himself unequal to the task of forming the league because he suffered a speech impediment. Hiawatha, however, was an imposing man with a fluent tongue. Together, in the time-honored fashion of a wise leader who relies on his executive assistant

to make his speeches, Dekanawida and Hiawatha might be effective in restoring sanity and peace to their nations.

Hiawatha was inspired. Tirelessly, the two men traveled up and down the land...Hiawatha fervently preaching the alliance outlined by Dekanawida.

Most Iroquois were at first hesitant to trust a plan that contained their enemies. Thadodaho, an Onondaga leader, relentlessly opposed Hiawatha. In a dramatic showdown, Hiawatha's superior spiritual power overcame the evil Thadodaho. Hiawatha combed out of Thadodaho's hair the snakes that had marked him as a fearful sorcerer.

Then the five nations—Mohawk, Oneida, Onondaga, Cayuga, and Seneca—came together, fifty great chiefs meeting in a grand council at the principal town, in the center of the alliance territory.[144]

Each of these men and women found a way to overcome stuttering, and this became the basis of his or her success. For each, their disability became their strength—and perhaps each looks back and sees stuttering as a gift.

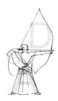

Stuttering Support Groups

Likely you've never met another stutterer. You've never seen a book about stuttering in a bookstore. You may be the first stutterer that your speech-language pathologist has met. You might feel that you're the only person in the world with this problem.

Last month your speech-language pathologist printed a webpage for you with the time and place of a stuttering support group. You put it off last month, but this month you go. You drive by the house. You see a group of people in the living room. You sit in your car, not sure if you have the courage to walk into the house.

Let's back up to how you find a stuttering support group. Call the National Stuttering Association at (800) 364-1677 or visit their website at http://www.nsastutter.org/. The NSA has more than 70 local support groups across the United States. Many stutterers say that the annual NSA convention is the best experience of their lives.

Speak Easy International has stuttering support groups in the New York-New Jersey area. Call Bob Gathman, at (201) 262-0895.

The National Association of Young People Who Stutter (866 866-8335, http://www.FriendsWhoStutter.org/) has support groups for children and teenagers who stutter.

Some speech clinics have their own stuttering support groups. These are often for practicing therapy. Practicing in a group is better than practicing alone.

If you're outside the United States, find a stuttering support organization in your country by visiting the International Stuttering Association website at http://www.stutterisa.org/.

Then there are the online support groups. Yahoo Groups (http://groups.yahoo.com/) lists more than seventy stuttering e-mail lists. The Usenet discussion group is alt.support.stuttering.

The online support groups tend to be a few individuals who do 90% of the chatting, and hundreds of people who don't write anything. One individual used several e-mail addresses and fake names to have long arguments with himself. After that, I set up a free database website, http://www.FriendshipCenter.com, where you can search for stutterers who share your age, occupation, religion, marital status, live near you, or a dozen other parameters. You can find the one person you want to talk to, rather than shotgunning an e-mail list.

Benefits of Support Groups

Cancer patients who joined a support group, without receiving treatment, lived longer than patients who received treatment, without a support group. In other words, support groups were more effective than surgery, drugs, or radiation in fighting cancer.

A support group will help you learn what works for other people. You'll get feedback on what you're doing. A group of people will generate new ideas that no individual would have thought of.

In a support group, you'll find that you've solved problems that other people face. Other people may have solved problems you face. Stuttering will no longer seem like one big problem, but rather will become a set of small problems.

When you ask your support group how to solve a small problem (e.g., answering the telephone at work) they'll tell you. If your support group has six members, you'll get six solutions to your problem. At least.

A support group improves your emotional state. Hearing other people's experiences improves your perspective. Your setbacks don't seem so bad. Sharing positive experiences makes everyone in the group feel good.

When you feel frustrated or depressed, you have no idea what to do. Talking to individuals who've been in the same situation will help you see that you have choices (see the section "Personal Construct Therapy," page 95).

Support Group Activities

I was a National Stuttering Association chapter leader. Our meetings usually had a dozen people. We met twice a month. One monthly meeting would have a guest speaker or activity. The other monthly meeting would for "sharing" (talking about personal experiences).

Guests and activities included:

- A speech-language pathologist who stuttered and was the superintendent of the county office of education. She was responsible for 33 school districts and seven community colleges.
- A filmmaker who stuttered showed us the roughcut of his documentary about stuttering. We were the first audience to see the video.
- Local speech-language pathologists presented their approaches to stuttering therapy.
- A psychologist presented his mind-body-spirit approach to stuttering treatment.
- Another psychologist, who stuttered, and was an expert in marital counseling, conducted a workshop on improving communications in relationships.
- A National Stuttering Association board member presented a paper he'd written about his philosophy of stuttering.
- We watched a video about Tourette's syndrome and discussed similarities to stuttering. (I was unable to find anyone with Tourette's to join us for that meeting.)
- When I couldn't find anyone else, I'd invite a Toastmasters International club. Those clubs are always have three or four people happy to make a speech about overcoming fear of making speeches!
- Short speeches about "What I did this summer."
- Reading Dr. Suess books in pairs. With choral speaking you don't stutter, although some of the Dr. Suess rhymes and made-up-words can trip you.

- Reading a Winnie-the-Pooh story with each character doing a type of speech therapy. Winnie-the-Pooh hums a lot, so he used continuous phonation. Owl used the Hot Airflow Method. Eeyore used Dreary Auditory Feedback, which is tediously slow and depressing, but makes you fluent. T-T-T-Tigger b-b-b-bounced his words. Rabbit talked fast, which makes you stutter. In contrast, the narrator read slowly.

- The funnest meeting was the Speech Disorders Game. I passed out large cards, each with a speech disorder: stuttering, lisping, aphasia (forgetting simple words), spastic dysphonia, speaking in a high voice, speaking in a low voice, speaking fast, speaking slow, unusual accents, spoonerisms (switching the first sounds of words, e.g., the academic toast "Let us glaze our asses to the queer old Dean"), etc. Each person introduced himself using his speech disorder, explaining what it was. Then the speech disorders became hearing disorders. In other words, the "lisp" person could only hear people who lisped, the "accent" person could only hear people who spoke in a funny accent. To carry on a conversation with several people, you had to constantly change your speech! People talked and talked and talked, for an hour, saying inane things to each other in funny voices. Or else they were laughing at other people. No one stuttered! Several people were astoundingly good at spoonerisms and hilarious accents. We also learned that there are worse speech disorders than stuttering.

Talking About Your Stuttering

One of my customers sent me this e-mail:

> I am a severe stutterer. At the time I ordered the Pocket DAF, I was blocking on every single word I spoke. I decided to try the DAF with the encouragement of my speech therapist.
>
> The first day I brought it to work, everyone in my of-

fice tried it. Before long, everyone in the entire office area was in my office wanting to hear me talk and try it out themselves.

I found the experience both wonderful and frightening. It was wonderful to know that so many of my co-workers wanted something good for me and were so excited about seeing it happening. It was frightening because I didn't know if the effects of the DAF would last. I've found that having the DAF allows (forces) me to be more open about my stuttering because everyone can see that I'm using some sort of device. I also think that it helps people understand my stuttering. If something analogous to a hearing aid can help, maybe my stuttering doesn't seem so mysterious to them after all!

After using the device over a year now, I'm very pleased to report that many people at the National Stuttering Project convention remarked on how much my fluency had improved since they last talked to me.

I use the DAF only sometimes at work and most of the time on the telephone. I'm very glad that I bought it.

In ten years working with the same people, she'd never discussed her speech. When she brought up the subject, she found that her co-workers wanted to support her.

Watch the video I made interviewing people about my speech. You'll see that everyone was supportive. (The video is on the DVD that comes with this book, or on my website.)

Listeners have different messages for mild and severe stutterers. Mild stuttering is "no big deal" or even appealing to listeners. A movie producer told me that my stuttering was appealing because it showed that I wasn't a "phony" person. Apparently she'd met plenty of "phony" people in Los Angeles (i.e., people who pretended to be someone they weren't).

In contrast, a mild stutterer may be able to successfully hide stuttering, but listeners figure out that he's hiding something. Listeners may not know what he is hiding, but he'll come across as "phony" or dishonest.

Listeners have a different message for severe stutterers. Severe stuttering disturbs listeners. They don't understand stuttering. They want to know if there's anything they can do to help you. But they're too polite to ask you about your disability. They want you to educate them. They don't want the proverbial "elephant in the living room" that no one will talk about.

The Disability Hierarchy

Some disabilities get more respect than others. Most people respect individuals with visible physical disabilities. For example, you'd make room on a crowded bus for a paraplegic using a wheelchair.

Individuals with non-visible physical disabilities, such as heart disease, get less respect. Would you give up your seat on a bus for a man who said that he had a heart condition and couldn't stand for long periods? What if he were your age and looked healthy?

Non-physical, visible disabilities get even less respect. For example, a man gets onto a bus, talking excitedly to no one. You don't see a cellphone earset in his ear. Plus he's repeating the same paranoid sentence over and over. You suspect he has schizophrenia. You see people on the bus getting up from their seats as he approaches—and getting off at the next stop.

The least respected disabilities are non-physical and non-visible. Stutterers look normal, until we talk. Listeners feel shock seeing you go from normal behavior one moment to head jerks, facial spasms, and being stuck in dysfluencies the next moment.

But you can move up the disability hierarchy. You can change your stuttering into a visible, physical disability:

- Wear a National Stuttering Association button.
- Tell people that you stutter.
- Tell a stuttering joke (page 115).
- Show people your anti-stuttering device.

In contrast, hiding your stuttering throws away the respect and support that people would otherwise give you.

I used to get calls asking for an anti-stuttering device that was completely invisible, 100% effective, and required no speech therapy. I'd explain that no stuttering treatment could do that. Then I'd suggest that perhaps their real problem wasn't stuttering, but rather was fear of listeners discovering that they stuttered. If you fear listeners discovering that you stutter, then your stress increases and you're more likely to stutter.

My company used to have a 10% return rate. Then another company marketed their anti-stuttering device as an invisible "miracle cure." Since then I've gotten no calls from stutterers wanting invisible instant cures. My return rate has dropped to less than 1%. I've heard that the other company has more than a 25% return rate. I'm happy that the "miracle cure" stutterers buy from them, not me.

What to Talk About

Of course, stuttering doesn't often come up as a topic of conversation. You'll have to bring it up.

I used to go up to strangers and say "My speech therapist wants me to introduce myself to more people..." That leads to listeners asking about speech therapy and stuttering.

Now I take my anti-stuttering device out of my pocket, and say that I'm putting on my anti-stuttering device. Almost always the listener asks me about the device.

I then ask the listener if she wants to try the device. I explain that I can adjust the device to make fluent people stutter.

Then all the conversations in the room stop. Everyone turns to watch my victim tripping over her tongue trying to count to ten with DAF adjusted to 200 milliseconds. Then they line up to try the device. And sometimes, after I've been the life of the party for a while, an attractive person wants to talk to me at length about stuttering, usually because she has a friend or relation who stutters.

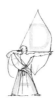

Stuttering at Work

I am 21 years old. Recently, I graduated from my third college course and still no job. Interviews come by the dozens but job offers are none! I am a Pharmacy Assistant Health Care Aide plus a medical transcriptionist, but after all the years in school and all the money spent on education, I am still unable to find work! Am I to live in poverty because people only see me at my worst?

Interviews for me are a horrid experience. I've had people pick up a newspaper and start reading it, waiting for me to get out of a block. All the interviewers act as if I'm wasting their time. It's more like they're wasting mine.

If people could only see me when I am fluent I'm sure I would have a job. On interviews I find myself apologizing for my speech...but why do I?

Is there anyone out there who is experiencing the same problems? I need help to cope.[145]

I am an embedded software engineer, and today I was faced with a situation that I have not run into yet in my pursuit of employment. Like many of you I have had the phone hung up on me by recruiters, or they rudely and quickly end the phone conversation. I had a personal phone interview with Motorola. First, the interview was designed to be very high stress. Second, the questions were given to me in advance which only made the situation worse. Of course it being a phone interview made it worst. I was unable to form sentences and completely locked up on the interview and was eliminated from the running for this software engineering position. Can I do anything? According to the recruiter I'm a great fit for the position, god this is frustrating.[146]

Graduate students in my stuttering class [surveyed employers, who] indicated that they would prefer to hire someone who was deaf or someone with moderate cerebral palsy rather than someone who stuttered. Interestingly, several of the employers who said they would not hire a stutterer had one or more stutterers already working for them.

When we probed to understand the WHY behind the employers' responses, we learned that essentially they thought they "understood" deafness and cerebral palsy, but stuttering was strange—and they assumed that persons who stutter were strange.[147]

Ten months after completing a stuttering therapy program, 44% of stutterers had received a promotion. 40% had changed jobs, 36% reporting that the change was for the better. Combining these, about 60% had improved employment after stuttering therapy. The study also found that 88% of the stutterers had maintained their fluency.

Their employers reported a 20% improvement in "communication effectiveness" for the stutterers completing therapy.[148]

Stutterers earn approximately $7200 less per year than non-stutterers.[149] Two groups of 25 persons were examined. The groups were matched for age, sex, IQ, race, education, and socioeconomic background. The subjects were contacted ten years after graduating from college. They were asked a number of questions relating to levels of achievement. The difference did not appear to be the result of employer discrimination. Rather, the stutterers were reluctant to accept promotions that involved making presentations to groups of people:

I have refused (or went "kicking") different projects at my job, which may/may not lead to promotions. Most recently, I went kicking on co-facilitating a corporate-wide quality workshop initiative. My partner in facilitation, after much coaxing by me, took the majority of the speaking sections, while I became her assistant. (Please be aware that I have not discussed my disorder with my co-workers, I am a mild stutterer that can usually "pass" for a fluent speaker.) I am now interested in changing careers and am looking for careers that focus on "behind the scenes" work...in other words, technical writing. I have considered such careers as Law, but have veered away from them.[150]

Talk About Your Stuttering

Another interview lasted about two minutes. The interviewer (another personnel director—they seem to be the worst problem) found an excuse to say I was not qualified for the job—so good-bye. I protested, asked for the technical interview and was asked to leave. As his excuse was plainly made up—this was also probably a case of discrimination.[151]

Begin the interview by talking about your stuttering. You may only get two minutes if you don't!

Whether you're looking for a job or already have a job, talk about your stuttering. Many people feel uncomfortable talking to a person who stutters. Educate them about stuttering to make them feel comfortable.

Some people make incorrect assumptions about individuals who stutter. For example, some people think that individuals who stutter are mentally retarded—even if you have a Ph.D.!

"Excellent communication skills" is the #1 qualification employers look for. Regardless of whether the help-wanted ad included this, say that you have excellent communication skills. Give concrete examples:

- If you're in a speech therapy program, discuss your progress and the techniques or strategies you use.
- If you learned nonavoidance skills in speech therapy, explain that although you stutter, you've overcome your fears of talking to strangers, etc.
- "I can say a phrase fluently if I say it a lot. In my last job, I

pretty much said the same things to customers all day, and my speech was fine." This should be acceptable for retail jobs, etc.

- If you use an electronic anti-stuttering device, show it to the interviewer and explain how it works.

- If the job requires making presentations, say that you can't say as much as non-stutterers so you prepare your remarks in advance and get right to the main points, unlike people who ramble on for half an hour.

Membership in Toastmasters proves that you have excellent communication skills. Toastmasters gives out lots of prizes, so mention if you won a blue ribbon for one of your speeches.

Communication is a two-way street. Say that you may not speak as well as other people, but you listen more carefully. Demonstrate that by not interrupting the interviewer, and by rephrasing and repeating back his questions. Ask the interviewer whether listening or speaking is more important in the job—they'll always say that listening is more important.

> The interview for the job that I currently have was one of the few interviews in which I discussed in depth the nature of my stuttering problem. I spent about a half-hour discussing my speech, and I think that it was very helpful for the interviewer in understanding how well I could work around my handicap.[152]

The Americans With Disabilities Act

In 1992, the Americans with Disabilities Act (ADA) outlawed employment discrimination against individuals with disabilities. Speaking was defined as a "major life activity" that the inability to do is disabling.

The central point of the ADA is that individuals with a disability can ask their employer (or potential employer) for a *reasonable accommodation*. A reasonable accommodation is a change to the job that will enable the individual to do the job. For example, a stutterer might ask that someone else answer the telephone. Or he might ask that the employer buy an anti-stuttering telephone.

When an individual with a disability requests a reasonable accommodation, the employer must make the accommodation. The individual must make the request. If the individual doesn't make such a request, the employer is not obligated to suggest an accommodation, or to hire the individual.

Employers aren't allowed to ask employees (or potential employees) about disabilities. You have to bring up the subject.

For more information about the ADA, visit the Equal Employment Opportunity Commission website at http://www.eeoc.gov or http://www.justice.gov/disabilities.htm.

The ADA does not apply to the federal government, including the military services. The ADA covers only employment discrimination. Other laws may cover discrimination or harassment outside of work (e.g., bad service in a restaurant).

Vocational Rehabilitation

If you're looking for a job, make an appointment with a vocational rehabilitation counselor. Look in your telephone directory's blue (government) pages under your state's department of labor.

Voc rehab counselors want you to succeed. They'll get you whatever therapy, anti-stuttering devices, or job training you need. The only complaint I've heard about voc rehab is the waiting lists. You may have to wait months to get help.

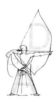

Listener Reactions

In 2003 I was in an acting class. We wrote, directed, and performed an original play. After the final performance a friend videotaped me asking audience members what they thought of me stuttering in the play. You can read the transcript below or watch the video on the DVD that comes with this book (the video is also on my website).

First Interview

WOMAN: I thought you did a great job. And at first I didn't know if it was part of the acting or not. I even asked Richard if it was part of it or not. I couldn't even tell if you were acting or if it was real. But I thought you did a great job and I didn't think it made it any worse than it would have been if you didn't stutter. I thought it was great.

Second Interview

WOMAN: I thought you were excellent. I met you before the show so I already knew. But it was like part of the act. I didn't know that was an anti-stutter device. I just thought that was part of your costume. I thought you were great.

Third Interview

TDK: What did you think of my stuttering?

MAN: It just seemed natural, like a part of who you were. And also there were times when you used it well.

TDK: If you heard that another play had an actor who stuttered in it, would that make you less likely to go see the play, or would you not care?

FAST-TALKING WOMAN: It gives the opportunity to slow down and actually the words that are being said. Otherwise if they're flying by too fast then it just kinda does just that, you're not even able to catch it as it rides by. But if you slow down and catch, you syllabalize it goes then that would seem to me to be a good thing. Just kinda slowing down the gears a little bit, snapping them back.

Fourth Interview
TDK: What did you think about me stuttering?

SETH'S MOM: Well, what I first thought that it was part of your act. Then eventually I caught on and I just thought it was great that you were performing and just being who you were and being an actor and making us all comfortable with that. It's not an experience I have every day, communicating with someone that has any kind of speech difficulties. And then the part where you said, "No, I just stutter," after the crushed nut episode, that was just a real, it just helped us all, kind of, yeah, it was a joke, and broke the ice, along with everything else being, talk about rawness of human emotions and kind of everything laid open, it was very helpful, and once again remembering that we're all human and we all have things to contribute and we all have things we don't like about us.

SETH: I felt like it's engaging to watch you perform because what's engaging about a performer is presence, and you're ability to stay present with the dynamic of your character, even though you're stuttering. It's very interesting, it's like, if you're that committed as a performer, to move through what might be difficult, it engages me.

TDK: What did you think of my electronic anti-stuttering device? Was it weird or distracting that I was using this?

SETH: Well, since I know you, David, I thought, OK, I wonder if that's an anti-stuttering device? But I didn't even think about that until I'd seen it like ten minutes into the show. It was just like, maybe this is character. I really that it was part of a shift of character because you used it really well.

TDK: There's a group of teenagers who stutter in New York City who've formed an acting company. Is there anything you'd like to tell them?

SETH: Hell yeah! I support you in training as young warrior artists.

Fifth Interview
TDK: What did you think about me stuttering?

DUNE: I just saw these different characters on stage, and it was just a quality of that character. Every different, completely different character. It took on a different quality, just like any other attribute that a person would have.

TDK: A group of teenagers who stutter in New York City have formed an acting company. Is there anything you'd like to say to them?

DUNE: Right on! Just keep doing what you're doing. I mean, I think that watching the performance, people that are trying out these different aspects of themselves, I want to do it. So I think that anyone that's doing it, go for it. It must be really a freeing thing, and takes a lot of courage.

Sixth Interview
TDK: Nir Banai was also in this play. What was it like working with a person who stuttered?

NIR BANAI: It was great. It was very inspiring to see you do such a performance with stuttering and having so much confidence to do it. It was really impressive. It was so impressive that you even used it as a joke in one of the skits. I was really impressed that you feel so comfortable with it.

Seventh Interview

TDK: If you heard that another actor in another play stuttered, would that make you less likely to go to the play?

MAN: Well, no, I don't think so. I mean, no. Definitely not.

TDK: There's a group of teenagers who stutter in New York who have formed an acting company. Is there anything you'd like to say to them?

MAN: Well, um, so, I think if they are looking for some inspiration then, um, well, if I was them I would have found that tonight.

Eighth Interview

TDK: What did you think about me stuttering?

GIGGLING WOMAN: I thought it was beautiful. You did a great job, I thought it was very real. Yeah, I was convinced—

TDK: Well, it was real, I do stutter!

GIGGLING WOMAN: You do stutter? No, you don't really stutter, do you?

TDK: Amazingly real, isn't it?

GIGGLING WOMAN: It was. It was very very real.

TDK: Wow. Great. I achieved that.

GIGGLING WOMAN: Yeah.

TDK: What did you think of the electronic anti-stuttering device I was wearing?

GIGGLING WOMAN: Oh this thing? I thought that was super cool. I did, I thought it was great.

Ninth Interview
TDK: What did you think of me stuttering?

WOMAN: It was beautiful. For real. I thought, I was much more, like, into the creativity of the play and thought that you guys pulled off a really beautiful creation, that you guys made.

TDK: You weren't wishing they had someone who wasn't stuttering?

WOMAN: No way, man. No way. I thought it was beautiful. It was great. You were great. I was very impressed.

Other Fluency Disorders

Cluttering

Cluttering (also called *tachyphemia*) is a communication disorder characterized by speech that is diffiicult for listeners to understand due to rapid speaking rate, erratic rhythm, poor syntax or grammar, and words or groups of words unrelated to the sentence. The person with cluttering may experience a short attention span, poor concentration, poorly organized thinking, inability to listen, and a lack of awareness that his or her speech is unintelligible.

Cluttering is sometimes confused with the stuttering. Both communication disorders break the normal flow of speech. However, stuttering is a speech disorder, whereas cluttering is language disorder. In other words, a stutterer knows what he or she wants to say, but can't say it; in contrast, a clutterer can say what he or she is thinking, but his or her thinking becomes disorganized during speaking.

Stutterers are usually dysfluent on initial sounds, when beginning to speak, and become more fluent towards the ends of utterances. In contrast, clutterers are most clear at the start of utterances, but their speaking rate increases and intelligibility decreases towards the end of utterances.

Stuttering is characterized by struggle behavior, such as overtense speech production muscles. Cluttering, in contrast, is effortless.

To compare, a stutterer trying to say "I want to go to the store," might sound like "I wa-wa-want to g-g-go to the sssssssssstore." In contrast, a clutterer might say, "I want to go to the st...uh...place where you buy...market st-st-store."

Cluttering is also characterized by slurred speech, especially dropped or distorted /r/ and /l/ sounds; and monotone speech that starts loud and trails off into a murmur.

Clutterers often also have reading and writing disorders, especially sprawling, disorderly handwriting, which poorly integrate ideas and space.

A clutterer described the feeling associated with a clutter as:

> It feels like 1) about twenty thoughts explode on my mind all at once, and I need to express them all, 2) that when I'm trying to make a point, that I just remembered something that I was supposed to say, so the person can understand, and I need to interrupt myself to say something that I should have said before, and 3) that I need to constantly revise the sentences that I'm working on, to get it out right.[153]

Another clutterer wrote on an Internet support group:

> I just seem to rush through the words, and often slur words together and/or mumble—and as a result I often have to slow down, concentrate, and repeat myself.

Because clutterers have poor awareness of their disorder, they may be indifferent or even hostile to speech-language pathologists. Treatment for cluttering usually takes longer than stuttering treatment. Delayed auditory feedback (DAF, see page 13) is usually used to produce a more deliberate, exaggerated oral-motor response pattern. Other treatment components include improving narrative structure with story-telling picture books, turn-taking practice, pausing practice, and language therapy.

Head Injuries and Strokes

Strokes and head injuries can cause repetitions, prolongations, and blocks. However, these *neurogenic* stutterers lack the struggle behavior and fears and anxieties of developmental stuttering.

Developmental stutterers can fluently speak certain memorized phrases, such as the "Pledge of Allegiance." Neurogenic stutterers are disfluent on everything. Developmental stutterers can speak fluently in certain (typically low-stress) situations. Neurogenic stutterers are disfluent everywhere.

Psychogenic Stuttering

Rarely, traumatic experiences cause an adult to start stuttering. *Psychogenic* stuttering usually involves rapid, effortless repetitions of initial sounds, without struggle behavior.

Spasmodic Dysphonia

This speech disorder is characterized by sudden involuntary movements of the vocal folds during speech. Some individuals have involuntary tightening of their vocal folds; others have involuntary relaxation; and still others have both. The resulting speech sounds either strained and strangled, or weak and breathy.

The disorder typically affects middle-aged persons, and affects more women than men. For more information see

http://en.wikipedia.org/wiki/Spasmodic_dysphonia

Social Anxiety Disorder

Individuals with this disorder experience fear and apprehension in social situations. For more information see

http://en.wikipedia.org/wiki/Social_anxiety

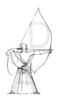

Recommended Books

Fun With Fluency: Direct Therapy with the Young Child, by Patty Walton and Mary Wallace (1998; ISBN: 1883315395) is the best book I've read about treating children ages two to seven years old. It's about *direct* stuttering therapy (page 125), without the old, ineffective *indirect* methods. Includes easy, stretchy speech; making direct requests for easy speech; modeling self-corrections; and playing speech games.

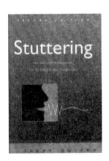

Stuttering: An Integrated Approach to Its Nature and Treatment, by Barry Guitar (1998; ISBN: 0683038001) is the best textbook about stuttering. The first part of the book presents the essentials of stuttering research. The second part of the book differentiates stuttering modification therapy from fluency shaping therapy, and then shows how to integrate the two therapies. The writing is clear and understandable.

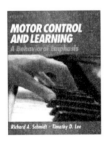

Motor Control and Learning: A Behavioral Emphasis, by Richard Schmidt and Tim Lee (2005; ISBN: 073604258X) is about how our brains learn and execute complex motor (muscle) skills (see page 28). If the stuttering "experts" were to read this book, stuttering therapy would advance fifty years.

Stuttering: A Life Bound Up In Words, by Marty Jezer (1997; ISBN: 0465081274). Jezer was a talented and entertaining writer, and author of a biography of Abbie Hoffman and other books. This is Jezer's autobiography, and stuttering affected everything in his life. You learn much about stuttering therapies, because Jezer went through just about every therapy program (and still stuttered).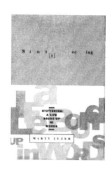

Knotted Tongues, by Benson Bobrick (1996; ISBN: 1568361211). The bulk of the book is about historical and literary persons who stuttered. These include Moses, Charles I, Lewis Carroll, Henry James, W. Somerset Maugham, and Winston Churchill. Bobrick also covers the history of stuttering treatments. The book also has a thirty-page overview of stuttering science, and a twenty-page overview of stuttering therapies.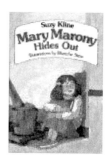

The *Mary Marony* series, by Suzy Kline, portrays a seven-year-old girl who stutters. She's supported by her parents, speech-language pathologist, and teacher. In *Mary Marony Hides Out* (1996; ISBN: 0440411351), Mary's favorite author comes to talk to her school, but Mary is afraid to speak to her so hides in the bathroom.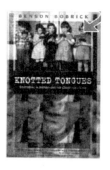

Practice Word Lists

These 357 words include every combination of consonant and vowel in the English language. The first column spells the sounds in the International Phonetic Alphabet.

Word List 1

e	able		
be	baby		
tße	chainsaw		
de	dateline		
fe	famous		
ge	gatepost		
he	halo		
dΩe	jaywalk		
ke	cable		
le	label		
me	mailbag		
ne	nadir	nay-deer	The lowest point
pe	pacer		
re	rabies		
se	saber	Cavalry sword	
ße	shapeless		
te	table		
∂e	they		
ve	vacant		
we	weightless		
„e	whale		
ze	zany		

175

Word List 2

æ	abbey	A monastery
bæ	baboon	
tßæ	chalice	
dæ	dancer	
fæ	famine	
gæ	gadget	
hæ	hacksaw	
dΩæ	jasmine	A climbing shrub with white flowers
kæ	cabin	
læ	ladder	
mæ	macro	
næ	knapsack	
pæ	package	
ræ	rabbit	
sæ	saddle	
ßæ	shadow	
tæ	tactile	
∂æ	than	
†æ	thankful	
væ	vanish	
wæ	wacky	
„æ	whacker	
jæ	yammer	
zæ	zander	European perch fish

Word List 3

å	achoo	
bå	baa	
tßå	cha-cha	
då	dachshund	
få	father	
gå	gaga	
hå	hah	
dΩå	jaunt	
kå	calf	
lå	launch	
må	macho	
nå	nachos	
på	pasta	
rå	rajah	Indian prince
så	psalm	
ßå	shah	Sovereign of Iran
tå	tabla	Indian hand drums
wå	waft	
jå	yahoo	Boorish or stupid person
Ωå	genre	

Word List 4

eager
beachfront
cheap
dealer
feature
geese
healer
genius
kiwi
legion
meager
kneecap
peaceful
react
cease-fire
sheepdog
teak
thee
theme
V-eight
weasel
wheel
yeast
zeal

Word List 5

any
bedtime
checkbook
dentist
felon
guest
health
gentle
kettle
leather
meadow
nephew
peck
redwood
self-talk
shepherd
ten-speed
them
theft
vent
wealthy
whether
yell
zest

Word List 6

aisle
byte
child
diamond
fiber
guide
height
jive
cayenne
lion
micro
knife
pie
rhino
cyclist
shiner
thyme
thy
thigh
vibrant
wildcat
whitefish
yipe
xylan (plant substance)

Word List 7

image
bemoan
chipmunk
divide
fishbowl
gift-wrap
hitchhike
ginger
kibbutz
lily
midcourse
nimble
picture
rebel
system
shiftless
ticket
this
thicket
vicar
wizard
whimsy
yip
zigzag

Word List 8

oaken
boastful
choke
domain
focus
ghost
hoagie (sandwich)
joke
coleslaw
locust
motion
noble
pollster
romance
soapstone
chauffer
toaster
those
thole (endure)
vogue
woven
yolk
zonal

Word List 9

otter
bobcat
chocolate
docile
foggy
goblin
hobby
jogger
cobbler
lobster
model
knockout
pocket
robin
soccer
shocker
toddler
volley
waffle
whopper
yacht

Word List 10

alder
bald
chalk
daughter
fallen
gauntlet
hallmark
jaunt
caller
laundry
mossy
gnaw
pause
raucous
salted
shawl
talking
thoughtful
vault
walker
yawn

Word List 11

onion
bubble
chubby
doesn't
fungus
govern
hovel
judge
color
love
money
knuckle
pump
rough
someday
shutter
touchdown
thus
thumbnail
vulgar
once
what
youngster

Word List 12

oil
boil
choice
doily   (small napkin)
foible
goiter
hoist
join
coin
loin
moist
noise
poignant
royal
soil
toil
voice
yoicks   (cry to encourage foxhounds)

Word List 13

alarm
balloon
debris
facade
galore
hallo   greeting
kazoo
lacrosse
macaw
patrol
ramose   ray-mose   composed of branches

Word List 13, continued

salon
chagrin
taboo
valise   suitcase
yapok   South American water opossum
jeté   zhah-tay   ballet jump from one foot to the other

Word List 14

ouster
bough
chow
downbeat   (conductor's downstroke on first beat of a measure)
foul
gauss   (measure of magnetism)
hound
jounce   (bounce, jolt)
couch
loud
mountain
noun
pouch
round
sow
shout
tout   (extravagant praise)
thou
thousand
vouch
wound   (as in string, not as in injury)
yowl   (cry of distress)
zounds   (a mild oath)

Word List 15

butte
deuce
feudal
gewgaw   (showy   trifle, bauble)
hewn
coupon
mule
neutral
pewter
tuba
view
whew

Word List 16

oomph
butcher
football
good
hoof
cookbook
lookout
nook
pudding
roof
soot
shook
took
wolf
whoops

Word List 17

oops
boomer
chew
deuce
food
goober (peanut)
hoop
juice
coolant
lunar
moon
nougat
poodle
rupee
sewage
shoe
tomb
woo
whoosh
U-boat
zoo

REFERENCES

[1] Johannes C. Ziegler , , Catherine Pech-Georgel , Florence George , F.-Xavier Alario, and Christian Lorenzi. "Deficits in speech perception predict language learning impairment," PNAS, September 27, 2005, vol. 102, no. 39, 14110-14115; http://www.pnas.org/cgi/content/abstract/102/39/14110

[2] Merzenich, M., Jenkins, W., Johnston, P., Schreiner, C., Miller, S., and Tallal, P. "Temporal Processing Deficits of Language-Learning Impaired Children Ameliorated by Training," *Science* vol. 271, January 5 1996, p.77-80.

[3] Brown, S., Ingham, R., Ingham, J., Laird, A., Fox, P. "Stuttered and fluent speech production: An ALE meta-analysis of functional neuroimaging studies," *Human Brain Mapping*, Volume 25, Issue 1, 2005, pages 105-117.

[4] Salmelin R, Schnitzler A, Schmitz F, Jancke L, Witte OW, Freund HJ. "Functional organization of the auditory cortex is different in stutterers and fluent speakers." *Neuroreport* 1998 July 13;9(10):2225-2229; Braun, A.R., Varga, M., Stager, S., Schulz, G., Selbie, S., Maisog, J.M., Carsom, R.E., Ludlow, C.L. "Atypical Lateralization of Hemispehral Activity in Developmental Stuttering: An H215O Positron Emission Tomography Study," in *Speech Production: Motor Control, Brain Research and Fluency Disorders*, edited by W. Hulstijn, H.F.M. Peters, and P.H.H.M. Van Lieshout, Amsterdam: Elsevier, 1997.

[5] "Superior temporal gyrus," Wikipedia, 2006 September 19, http://en.wikipedia.org/wiki/Superior_temporal_gyrus.

[6] "Operculum (brain)," Wikipedia, 2006 September 19, http://en.wikipedia.org/wiki/Operculum_%28brain%29.

[7] Brown, S., Ingham, R., Ingham, J., Laird, A., Fox, P. "Stuttered and fluent speech production: An ALE meta-analysis of functional neuroimaging studies," *Human Brain Mapping*, 25(1), 2005, 105-117.

[8] Ibid.

[9] Kelly, Ellen. "Orofacial Muscle Activity of Children Who Stutter," *et al., Journal of Speech and Hearing Research*, 38:5, October 1995.

[10] Proctor A., Duff, M.. and Yairi, E. (2002). "Early childhood stuttering: African Americans and European Americans." *ASHA Leader*, 4:15, page 102.

[11] Craig. A, Hancock K, Tran. Y, Craig. M, & Peters, K. (2002). "Epidemiology of stuttering in the communication across the entire

life span." *Journal of Speech Language Hearing Research*, 45:1097-1105.

[12] http://www.stuttering.org/alumni.html

[13] Kutscher, Martin L. *Kids in the Syndrome Mix* (Jessica Kingsley Publishers, 2005, ISBN 1-84310-8100), pages 178-179.

[14] Braun, A.R., Varga, M., Stager, S., Schulz, G., Selbie, S., Maisog, J.M., Carsom, R.E., Ludlow, C.L. "Atypical Lateralization of Hemispehral Activity in Developmental Stuttering: An H215O Positron Emission Tomography Study," in *Speech Production: Motor Control, Brain Research and Fluency Disorders*, edited by W. Hulstijn, H.F.M. Peters, and P.H.H.M. Van Lieshout, Amsterdam: Elsevier, 1997.

[15] Watkins, K., S. Davis, P. Howell. "Brain activity during altered auditory feedback: an fMRI study in persistent and recovered developmental stuttering," Oxford Dysfluency Conference (2005), http://www.speech.psychol.ucl.ac.uk/conferences/WRKSHP05/watkins/watkins%20et%20al.doc

[16] Foundas, A.L., Bollich, A.B., Corey, D.M., Hurley, M., Heilman, K.M. "Anomalous Anatomy in Adults with Persistant Developmental Stuttering: A Volumetric MRI Study of Cortical Speech-Language Areas," *Neurology*, 2001 57:207-215.

[17] A. L. Foundas, MD, A. M. Bollich, PhD, J. Feldman, MD, D. M. Corey, PhD, M. Hurley, PhD, L. C. Lemen, PhD and K. M. Heilman, MD. "Aberrant auditory processing and atypical planum temporale in developmental stuttering," *Neurology*, 2004;63:1640-1646.

[18] Kalinowski, J., Armson, J., Stuart, A., Graco, V., and Roland-Mieskowski, M. "Effects of alterations in auditory feedback and speech rate on stuttering frequency," *Language and Speech, 1993*, 36, 1-16; Sark, S., Kalinowski, J., Stuart, A., Armson, J. "Stuttering amelioration at various auditory feedback delays and speech rates," *European Journal of Disorders of Communication, 31*, 259-269, 1996; Brenaut, L., Morrison, S., Kainowski, J., Armson, J., Stuart, A. "Effect of Altered Auditory Feedback on Stuttering During Telephone Use," Dalhousie University, Halifax, Nova Scotia, Canada, 1995; Stager, S., Denman, D., Ludlow, C. "Modifications in Aerodynamic Variables by Persons Who Stutter Under Fluency-Evoking Conditions." *Journal of Speech, Language, and Hearing Research, 40*, 832-847, August 1997. Zimmerman, S., Kalinowski, J., Stuart, A., Rastatter, M. "Effect of Altered Auditory Feedback on People Who Stutter During Scripted Telephone Conversations." *Journal of Speech, Language, and Hearing Research, 40*, 1130-1134, October 1997.

[19] Sark, S., Kalinowski, J., Stuart, A., Armson, J. "Stuttering amelioration at various auditory feedback delays and speech rates," *European Journal of Disorders of Communication*, 31, 259-269, 1996.

[20] Sark, S., Kalinowski, J., Stuart, A., Armson, J. "Stuttering amelioration at various auditory feedback delays and speech rates," *European Journal of Disorders of Communication*, 31, 259-269, 1996.

[21] Van Borsel, J., Reunes, G., Van den Bergh, N. "Delayed auditory feedback in the treatment of stuttering: clients as consumers," *International Journal of Language and Communication Disorders*, 2003, 38:2, 119–129.

[22] Radford, N., Tanguma, J., Gonzalez, M., Nericcio, M.A., Newman, D. "A Case Study of Mediated Learning, Delayed Auditory Feedback, and Motor Repatterning to Reduce Stuttering," *Perceptual and Motor Skills*, 2005, 101, 63-71.

[23] Ryan, B.P., Van Kirk, B. "The Establishment, Transfer and Maintenance of Fluent Speech in 50 Stutterers Using Delayed Auditory Feedback and Operant Procedures." *Journal of Speech and Hearing Disorders, 39*:1, February, 1974.

[24] Ryan, Bruce and Barbara Van Kirk Ryan. "Programmed Stuttering Treatment for Children: Comparison of Two Establishment Programs Through Transfer, Maintenance, and Follow-Up," *Journal of Speech and Hearing Research, 38*:1, February 1995.

[25] Elman, J. (1981). "Effects of frequency-shifted feedback on the pitch of vocal productions," *Journal of the Acoustical Society of America, 70* (1). Burnett, T.A., Senner, J.E., and Larson, C.R. (1997). "Voice F0 responses to pitch-shifted auditory feedback: A preliminary study," *J. Voice, 11*, 202-211. Burnett, T.A., Freedland, M.B., Larson, C.R., Hain, T.C. (1998). "Voice F0 responses to manipulations in pitch feedback," *Journal Acoustical Society of America, 103* (6) June 1998.

[26] Natke, U., Grosser, J., & Kalveram, K.Th. (2001) Fluency, fundamental frequency, and speech rate under frequency shifted auditory feedback in stuttering and nonstuttering persons. *Journal of Fluency Disorders*, 26, 227-241.

[27] Skotko, Janet. Special Interest Division 4 discussion group SID4@LISTSERV.TEMPLE.EDU, 2006 May 25.

[28] Stuart, A., Kalinowski, J., Rastatter, M., Saltuklaroglu, T., Dayalu, V. "Investigations of the impact of altered auditory feedback in-the-ear devices on the speech of people who stutter: initial fitting and 4-month follow-up," *International Journal of Language and Communication Disorders*, 2004, 39:1, 93–113.

[29] Runyan, Charles, and Sara E. Runyan. "The Speech Easy: A Two Year Study," presentation at the American Speech-Language Hearing Association convention, November 2005.

[30] Hyde, L. (2003). "Comparison of the [brand name deleted] and Casa Futura/Jabra fluency devices," presentation to the Canadian Association of Persons who Stutter conference, August 2003.

[31] Stuart, A., Xia, S., Jiang, Y., Jiang, T., Kalinowski, J., Rastatter, M. "Self-contained in-the-ear device to deliver altered auditory feedback: applications for stuttering," *Annals of Biomedical Engineering*, 31, 233-237, 2003.

[32] Stuart, A., Kalinowski, J., and Rastatter, M. (1997). Effect of monaural and binaural altered auditory feedback on stuttering frequency, *Journal of the Acoustical Society of America*, 111, 2237-2241.

[33] Stuart, A., Kalinowski, J., Armson, J., Stenstrom, R., and Jones, K. (1996). Stuttering reduction under frequency-altered feedback of plus and minus one-half and one-quarter octaves at two speech rates. *Journal of Speech and Hearing Research*, 39, 396-401.

[34] America Wins Olympics, October 2, 2000, http://truthnews.net/culture/2000_10_olympic.html

[35] Arielle Ford's Complete Book Publicity Workshop.

[36] Stager, S., Denman, D., Ludlow, C. "Modifications in Aerodynamic Variables by Persons Who Stutter Under Fluency-Evoking Conditions." *Journal of Speech, Language, and Hearing Research*, Volume 40, 832-847, August 1997.

[37] Boberg, E., & Kully, D. (1994). "Long-term results of an intensive treatment program for adults and adolescents who stutter." *Journal of Speech and Hearing Research*, 37, 1050-1059.

[38] Craig, A., et al. "A Controlled Clinical Trial for Stuttering in Persons Aged 9 to 14 Years" Journal of Speech and Hearing Research, 39:4, 808-826, August 1996. Hancock, et al. "Two- to Six-Year Controlled-Trial Stuttering Outcomes for Children and Adolescents," Journal of Speech and Hearing Research, 41:1242-1252, December 1998.

[39] Craig, A., Calver, P. "Following Up on Treated Stutterers: Studies of Perceptions of Fluency and Job Status." *Journal of Speech and Hearing Research*, 34, 279-284, April 1991.

[40] Onslow, M., et al., "Speech Outcomes of a Prolonged-Speech Treatment for Stuttering," *Journal of Speech and Hearing Research*, 39, 734-749, 1996.

[41] Ramig, P., Adams, M. Vocal changes in stutterers and nonstutterers during high- and low-pitched speech, *Journal of Fluency Disorders*, Volume 6, Issue 1, March 1981, Pages 15-33

[42] Elman, J. (1981). "Effects of frequency-shifted feedback on the pitch of vocal productions," *Journal of the Acoustical Society of America*, 70 (1). Burnett, T.A., Senner, J.E., and Larson, C.R. (1997). "Voice F0 responses to pitch-shifted auditory feedback: A preliminary study," J. Voice, 11, 202-211. Burnett, T.A., Freedland, M.B., Larson, C.R., Hain, T.C. (1998). "Voice F0 responses to manipulations in pitch feedback," *Journal of the Acoustical Society of America*, 103 (6) June 1998.

[43] Natke, U., & Kalveram, K.Th. (2001) Fundamental frequency and vowel duration under frequency shifted auditory feedback in stuttering and nonstuttering adults. In H.-G. Bosshardt, J. S. Yaruss & H. F. M. Peters (Eds.), Fluency Disorders: Theory, Research, Treatment and Self-help. Proceedings of the Third World Congress of Fluency Disorders in Nyborg, Denmark. Nijmegen: Nijmegen University Press, 66-71. Natke, U., Grosser, J., & Kalveram, K.Th. (2001) Fluency, funda-

mental frequency, and speech rate under frequency shifted auditory feedback in stuttering and nonstuttering persons. Journal of Fluency Disorders, 26, 227-241.

[44] Kottke, F.J., Halpern, D., Easton, J.K.M., Ozel, A.T., Burrill, C.A. "The Training of Coordination." *Archives of Physical Medicine and Rehabilitation*, Vol 59, December 1978, 567-572.

[45] Yamada Shoji. "The Myth of Zen in the Art of Archery," *Japanese Journal of Religious Studies*, 2001, 28/1-2; http://www.nanzan-u.ac.jp/SHUBUNKEN/ publications/jjrs/pdf/586.pdf

[46] Caruso, A., et al. "Adults Who Stutter: Responses to Cognitive Stress." *Journal of Speech and Hearing Research, 37*, 746-754, August 1994.

[47] Perkins, W., Dabul, B. "The Effects of Stuttering on Systolic Blood Pressure." *Journal of Speech & Hearing Research*, 16 (4), Dec 1973.

[48] Schwartz, Martin. Personal correspondence.

[49] Kuehn, Donald (1994). Official correspondence from the National Institute of Deafness and Communication Disorders (NIDCD).

[50] Bloodstein, Oliver (1995) *A Handbook On Stuttering,* 5th edition, San Diego: Singular Press.

[51] Bloodstein, Oliver (1996) "Stuttering as an Anticipatory Struggle Reaction," in R. F. Curlee & G. M. Siegel, *Nature and Treatment of Stuttering: New Directions.* Boston: Allyn&Bacon.

[52] Neiders, Gunars. Stutt-x e-mail correspondence, December 18, 1997.

[53] Prins, D., Madelkorn, T., Cerf, A. "Principal and Differential Effects of Haloperidol and Placebo Treatments Upon Speech Disfluencies in Stutterers." *Journal of Speech & Hearing Research, 23*, 614-629, September 1980.

[54] Stager, Ludlow, Gordon, Cotelingam, and Rapoport. "Fluency Changes in Persons Who Stutter Following a Double Blind Trial of Clomipramine and Desipramine," *Journal of Speech and Hearing Research*, June 1995.

[55] Goleman, Daniel, and Joel Gurin. *Mind/Body Medicine*, Consumer Reports Books, 1993.

[56] Brown, Walter A. "The Placebo Effect." *Scientific American*, January 1998, 90-96.

[57] Bloodstein, Oliver (1995) *A Handbook On Stuttering,* 5th edition, San Diego: Singular Press.

[58] Newman-Tancredi, Adrian. "Noradrenaline and adrenaline are high affinity agonists at dopamine D4 receptors." *European Journal of Pharmacology* 319 (1997) 379-383. 101511,274@compuserve@com. Valerie Audinot-Bouchez, Alain Gobert, Mark J. Millan, Department of Psychopharmacology, Institut de Recherches, 125 Chemin de Ronde, 78290 Croissy-sur-Seine (Paris), France.

[59] Bloodstein, Oliver (1995) *A Handbook On Stuttering,* 5th edition, San Diego: Singular Press.

[60] Caruso, A., *et al.* "Adults Who Stutter: Responses to Cognitive Stress." *Journal of Speech and Hearing Research, 37*, 746-754, August 1994.

[61] Kelly, George. *The Psychology Of Personal Constructs,* (Routledge, 1955, ISBN 0415037980).

[62] Clausen, Kjartan. The Aikido FAQ. March 8, 2002 http://www.aikidofaq.com/

[63] Andrews, G., Cutler, J. "Stuttering Therapy: The relation between changes in symptom level and attitudes." *Journal of Speech and Hearing Disorders, 39,* 312-319, 1974.

[64] Guitar, B. & Bass, C. (1978). "Stuttering therapy: The relation between attitude change and long-term outcome." *Journal of Speech and Hearing Disorders, 43,* 392-400.

[65] Comings, D., et al., "Polygenic Inheritance of Tourette Syndrome, Stuttering, Attention Deficit Hyperactivity, Conduct, and Oppositional Defiant Disorder," *American Journal of Medical Genetics 67*:264-288 (1996).

[66] Maguire, G., Riley, G.D., Wu, J.C., Franklin, D.L., Potkin, S. "Effects of risperidone in the treatment of stuttering," in *Speech Production: Motor Control, Brain Research and Fluency Disorders*, edited by W. Hulstijn, H.F.M. Peters, and P.H.H.M. Van Lieshout, Amsterdam: Elsevier, 1997.

[67] Riley, Glyndon. "Medical Aspects Of Stuttering," *Stuttering Foundation Of America* newsletter, Summer 2002.

[68] Gottlieb, Jeff. "Easier for Him to Say," *Los Angeles Times*, April 3, 2002.

[69] Stager, S., Calis, K., Grothe, D., Bloch, M., Turcasso, N., Ludlow, C., Braun, A. "A Double-Blind Trial of Pimozide and Paroxetine For Stuttering," in *Speech Production: Motor Control, Brain Research and Fluency Disorders*, edited by W. Hulstijn, H.F.M. Peters, and P.H.H.M. Van Lieshout, Amsterdam: Elsevier, 1997.

[70] Rothenberger, A., Johannsem, H., Schulze, H., Amorosa, H., Rommel, D. "Use of Tiapride on Stuttering in Children and Adolescents," *Perceptual and Motor Skills*, 1994, 79, 1163-1170.

[71] "Pagoclone," Indeveus Pharmaceuticals, 2006 June 11 http://www.indevus.com/product/pagaclone.asp?page=pagaclone

[72] Harkness, Richard, November 18, 2005, personal correspondence.

[73] Butcher, S. Stut-hlp posting, January 27, 1998. Reprinted with permission.

[74] Boberg, Julia. Institute for Stuttering Research and Treatment, Edmonton, Alberta. Reprinted with permission.

[75] Bloodstein, Oliver (1995) *A Handbook On Stuttering*, 5th edition, San Diego: Singular Press.

[76] Ibid.

[77] Ibid.

[78] Ibid.

[79] Ibid.

[80] De Nil, L., & Kroll, R. "The Relationship Between Locus of Control and Long-Term Stuttering Treatment Outcome in Adult Stutterers," *Journal of Fluency Disorders*, 20:4, December 1995.

[81] *Psychology Today*, November/December, 1998.

[82] Mitzman, David. "The Right Message," National Stuttering Association conference schedule, June 2006, page 26.

[83] Farber, Barry. *How to Learn Any Language*. 1991, ISBN 0-8065-1271-7, pages 97-98.

[84] Yairi, E., Ambrose, N. "Onset of stuttering in preschool children: Selected factors," *Journal of Speech and Hearing Research*, 35, 1992, 782-788.

[85] Yairi, E. (1993) "Epidemiologic and other considerations in treatment efficacy research with preschool-age children who stutter," *Journal of Fluency Disorders*, *18*, 197-220. Yairi, E., Ambrose, N. "Onset of stuttering in preschool children: Selected factors," *Journal of Speech and Hearing Research*, *35*, 1992, 782-788.

[86] Finn, Patrick. "Children Recovered From Stuttering Without Formal Treatment: Perceptual Assessment of Speech Normalcy," *Journal of Speech, Language, and Hearing Research*, 40, 867-876, August 1997.

[87] Andrews, et al., "Stuttering: a review of research findings and theories," *Journal of Speech and Hearing Disorders*, *48*, 226-246, 1983.

[88] Yairi, E, & Ambrose, N. (2005). *Early childhood stuttering*. Austin, TX: Pro-Ed, Inc. Kloth, S., Janssen, P., Kraaimaat, F. & Brutten, G. (1995). "Speech-motor and linguistic skills of young stutterers prior to onset." *Journal of Fluency Disorders*, 20, 157-170.

[89] Yairi, 2005; "On the Gender Factor in Stuttering," Stuttering Foundation of America newsletter, Fall 2005, page 5.

[90] Craig, et al., 2002; Craig, A. Tran, Y., Craig, M., & Peters, K. (2002). "Epidemiology of stuttering in the communication across the entire life span." *Journal of Speech, Language, and Hearing Research*, 45, 1097-1105.

[91] *ADVANCE For Speech-Language Pathologists*, July 6, 1998, page 22

[92] Nippold, M., Rudzinski, M. "Parents' Speech and Children's Stuttering: A Critique of the Literature," *Journal of Speech and Hearing Research*, *38*:5, October 1995.

[93] Meyers, S.C., & Freeman, F.J. (1985a) "Are mothers of stutterers different? An investigation of social-communicative interaction." *Journal of Fluency Disorders*, *10*, 193-209.

[94] Weiss, A.L., & Zebrowski, P.M. (1992) "Disfluencies in the conversations of young children who stutter: Some answers about questions." *Journal of Speech and Hearing Research*, 35, 1230-1238.

[95] Kelly, E.M. & Conture, E.G. (1992) "Speaking rates, response time latencies, and interrupting behaviors of young stutterers, non-stutterers, and their mothers." *Journal of Speech and Hearing Re-*

search, 37, 1256-1267; Kelly, E.M. (1994) "Speech rates and turn-taking behaviors of children who stutter and their fathers." *Journal of Speech and Hearing Research, 37*, 1284-1294; Yaruss, J.S., Conture, E.G. (1995) "Mother and Child Speaking Rates and Utterance Lengths in Adjacent Fluent Utterances: Preliminary Observations," *Journal of Fluency Disorders, 20*, 257-278; Yaruss, J.S. (1997) "Utterance Timing and Childhood Stuttering," *Journal of Fluency Disorders, 22*, 263-286.

[96] Howell, P., Kapoor, A, Rustin, L. "The Effects of Formal and Casual Interview Styles on Stuttering Incidence," in *Speech Production: Motor Control, Brain Research and Fluency Disorders*, edited by W. Hulstijn, H.F.M. Peters, and P.H.H.M. Van Lieshout, Amsterdam: Elsevier, 1997.

[97] Rommel, D., Häge, A., Johannsen, H., Schulze, H. "Linguistic Aspects of Stuttering In Childhood," in *Speech Production: Motor Control, Brain Research and Fluency Disorders*, edited by W. Hulstijn, H.F.M. Peters, and P.H.H.M. Van Lieshout, Amsterdam: Elsevier, 1997.

[98] Meyers, S.C., & Freeman, F.J. (1985b) "Interruptions as a variable in stuttering and disfluency." *Journal of Speech and Hearing Research, 28*, 428-435.

[99] Meyers, S.C., & Freeman, F.J. (1985c) "Mother and child speech rates as a variable in stuttering and disfluency." *Journal of Speech and Hearing Research, 28*, 436-444.

[100] Stephenson-Opsal, D., & Bernstein Ratner, N. (1988) "Maternal speech rate modification and childhood stuttering." *Journal of Fluency Disorders, 13*, 49-56.

[101] Meyers, S.C. (1990) "Verbal behaviors of preschool stutterers and conversational partners: Observing reciprocal relationships." *Journal of Speech and Hearing Disorders, 54*, 706-712.

[102] Kloth, S.A.M., Jannsen, P., Kraaimaat, F.W., Brutten, G.J. (1995) "Communicative Behavior of Mothers of Stuttering and Nonstuttering High-Risk Children Prior to the Onset of Stuttering," *Journal of Fluency Disorders, 20*, 365-377.

[103] Gladwell, Malcolm. "Do Parents Matter?" *The New Yorker*, August, 17, 1998, reviewing *The Nurture Assumption: Why Children Turn Out the Way They Do*, by Judith Rich Harris, 1998, ISBN 0684857073.

[104] Mary Wallace and Patty Walton, *Fun With Fluency: Direct Therapy With The Young Child* (Imaginart, 1998).

[105] Yairi, E, & Ambrose, N. (2005). *Early childhood stuttering*. Austin, TX: Pro-Ed, Inc. Kloth, S., Janssen, P., Kraaimaat, F. & Brutten, G. (1995). "Speech-motor and linguistic skills of young stutterers prior to onset. *Journal of Fluency Disorders, 20*, 157-170.

[106] Yairi, 2005; "On the Gender Factor in Stuttering," Stuttering Foundation of America newsletter, Fall 2005, page 5.

[107] Craig, et al., 2002; Craig, A. Tran, Y., Craig, M., & Peters, K. (2002). "Epidemiology of stuttering in the communication across the entire life span." *Journal of Speech, Language, and Hearing Research, 45*, 1097-1105.

[108] Craig, A., et al. "A Controlled Clinical Trial for Stuttering in Persons Aged 9 to 14 Years," *Journal of Speech and Hearing Research*, 39:4, 808-826, August 1996.

[109] Hancock, et al. "Two- to Six-Year Controlled-Trial Stuttering Outcomes for Children and Adolescents," *Journal of Speech and Hearing Research*, 41:1242-1252, December 1998.

[110] Kalinowski, J., Saltuklaroglu, T., Dayalu, V., Guntupalli, V. "Is it possible for speech therapy to improve upon natural recovery rates in children who stutter?" *International Journal of Language and Communication Disorders*, 40(3) 349-358.

[111] Brenner, Marie. "I Never Sang For My Mother." *Vanity Fair, 58*, August 1995, p.128.

[112] Nefsky, Art. Letter from Mel Tillis, Sept. 30, 1997, http://www.nefsky.com/tillis.htm

[113] Jones, James Earl. *Voice and Silences*, 1993.

[114] Drew, Polly. "A Stutter Won't Stop You," *Milwaukee Journal-Sentinal*, July 27, 1997, p.4L.

[115] Lawrence, M. "A Man of Many Words." *Sports Illustrated*, v79, n18, November 1, 1993, p.91.

[116] Reprinted with permission from the Stuttering Foundation of America newsletter, Spring/Summer 1996.

[117] *Ghostwriter*, 1993 (PBS drama series focused on illiteracy).

[118] Bobrick, Benson. *Knotted Tongues*. Simon&Schuster, 1995

[119] Gross, Terry. *Fresh Air*, August 15, 2000.

[120] Interviewed on National Public Radio's *All Things Considered*.

[121] Bobrick, Benson. *Knotted Tongues*. Simon&Schuster, 1995

[122] *Stuttering Foundation of America* newsletter, Summer 2002.

[123] Wallichenski, David. *Book of Lists* (Boston: Little, Brown, 1995); Fonzi, Gaeton. *Annenberg*. New York: Weybright & Talley, 1969; Toch, Thomas, "One man's gift to public education." *U.S. News & World Report*, November 1, 1993, v115, n17, p20.

[124] Zimmerman, I. "Photography That Speaks Volumes" *ADVANCE For Speech-Language Pathologists and Audiologists*, 7:50, March 23, 1998, page 22.

[125] Wolfe, Tom. *The Right Stuff.*

[126] ASHA Leader

[127] Richard Benyo, personal correspondance.

[128] Stuttering Foundation of America.

[129] Sculley, John. *Odyssey* (1987). p.111.

[130] Carlton, Jim. *Apple: The Inside Story of Intrigue, Egomania, and Business Blunders*. (New York: Random House, 1997).

[131] Weiner, Tim. "Sidney Gottlieb, 80, Dies; Took LSD to C.I.A." *New York Times*, March 10, 1999.

[132] Fraser, Antonia. *King James VI of Scotland, I of England*. (London: Weidenfeld and Nicolson; 1974) p. 163.

[133] Bobrick, Benson. *Knotted Tongues*. Simon&Schuster, 1995

[134] Ibid.

[135] Ibid.

[136] Montalbo, Thomas. "Churchill: A Study in Oratory," *Finest Hour*, 69, and The Churchill Centre (http://www.winstonchurchill.org/).

[137] Bobrick, Benson. *Knotted Tongues*. Simon&Schuster, 1995

[138] Ibid.

[139] Ian Hamilton, "An Oxford Union," *The New Yorker*, February 19, 1996.

[140] http://www.logophilia.com/waw/Campbell-Patrick.asp

[141] Exodus 4:10-17, *The New Oxford Annotated Bible, Revised Standard Edition*, 1973.

[142] Bobrick, Benson. *Knotted Tongues*. Simon&Schuster, 1995

[143] Ibid.

[144] Kehoe, Alice. *North American Indians: A Comprehensive Account*, 3rd edition, page 227. Prentice-Hall, Inc. (Englewood Cliffs, NJ), 1992. See also *Hiawatha and the Iroquois Confederation* and *Proc. of the American Association for the Advancement of Science* 30:324-341, both by Horatio E. Hale, 1882; and "Hi-a-wat-ha," by William M. Beauchamp, *Journal of American Folklore* 4(15):295-306, 1891.

[145] Giret, Karen. *Letting GO*, National Stuttering Association newsletter, July/August 1996.

[146] Possibly e-mail from STUTT-L.

[147] Freeman, Frances. 1993. University of Texas, personal correspondence.

[148] Craig, A., Calver, P. "Following Up on Treated Stutterers: Studies of Perceptions of Fluency and Job Status." *Journal of Speech and Hearing Research, 34*, 279-284, April 1991.

[149] Schwartz, Martin, 1996b. National Center for Stuttering website.

[150] Personal e-mail.

[151] David Bertollo, e-mail.

[152] Tom Morrow, e-mail.

[153] Reyes-Alami, C., "Interview with a Person who Clutters," 2004 March 3, http://www.mnsu.edu/comdis/kuster/cluttering/camil.html.

INDEX

A

adrenaline, 81
alcohol, 106
Americans with Disabilities
    Act, 163, 164
anxiety, 102, 104, 105
articulation, 120
attention deficit hyperactivity
    disorder, 100, 103, 133
avoidance, 8, 106, 121

B

beginning stuttering, 120
botulinum toxin, 105
brain, 6, 62, 100, 122, 133

C

CAFET, 136
Canada, 106
cerebral, 161
childhood stuttering, 2, 3, 8, 68,
    103, 120, 122, 125, 126, 128,
    130, 132, 134, 135, 139, 141,
    149, 185
cluttering, 170
cognitive, 39, 82
complexity, 106
computers, 3, 82, 98

D

delayed auditory feedback, 171
diaphragm, 6

dopamine, 65, 81, 100–104, 122

E

Effexor, 104
electronic devices, 130
embarrassment, 70, 121
employment, 160, 161, 163, 164
environmental cueing, 120

F

Fraser, Malcolm, 69

G

gentle onset, 46

H

haloperidol, 101
Harkness, Richard, 103
Herrigel, Eugen, 71–75

I

insurance, 132, 135
intensity, 102, 137
Internet, 102, 103

J

jaw, 7, 8, 81
Johnson, Wendall, 69
journals, 185

K

Kelly, 185

L

language, 70, 99, 132–134, 171
larynx, 6–8, 120
lips, 7, 8, 81
listeners, 3, 8, 50, 70

M

mentally-retarded, 3, 162
motor learning theory, 62
motor skills, 39

N

National Stuttering Association, 99
neurotransmitters, 100

O

obsessive-compulsive disorder (OCD), 100
olanzapine, 102

P

parents, 126, 130, 132–137
Personal Construct Therapy, 90, 95, 97, 154
phonation, 6, 8, 120
phonology, 133
Pimozide, 102
pitch, 120
placebos, 80
prolongations, 120, 121
Propanolol, 105
Prozac, 104
psychology, 107
public speaking, 70, 97, 99, 142, 147

R

repetitions, 120, 121

respiration, 6, 7, 71, 72, 81, 102, 120
Risperdal, 102
Ritalin, 103

S

serotonin, 104
speaking circles, 99
stress, 77, 80–82, 136, 160
stretched vowels, 126, 130
Stuttering Foundation of America, 69
substitutions, 8, 121
support groups, 97, 153

T

teenage stuttering, 136, 137
telephones, 98, 121, 163, 164
Tiapride, 102
Toastmasters International, 99, 163
tongue, 7, 8, 81, 120, 133, 147, 149, 151
Trazadone, 104

V

Van Riper, Charles, 70
vocal folds, 6, 7, 72, 73, 105
vocational rehabilitation, 164

W

Wellbutrin, 104
whispering, 7

Z

Zen, 69, 70, 74
Zoloft, 104
Zyprexa, 102